Entrust your works to the Lord and your plan will succeed.

Proverbs 16:3

Table of Contents

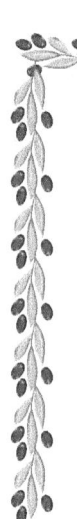

Dedication

My mom and I share a very special relationship. We actually like each other as well as love each other.

My mom has supported and encouraged me in every endeavor I have undertaken. She has inspired me in more ways than I can list here. The older I get the more clear is my understanding of the many lessons she has taught me about the importance of family, friends, generosity, thoughtfulness and perseverance.

Thank you, mom.

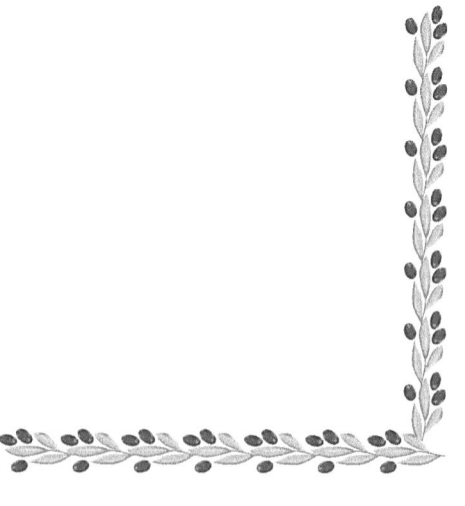

Introduction

I am not a doctor, nutritionist, counselor or any other type of trained professional. My rubber has met the road by way of 40 years of fighting my own obesity. In fourth grade, I heard the nuns commenting that I was already at the weight of a high school student. As an adult I suffered the humiliation of being unable to fit behind the wheel of a rented car (in front of a colleague) and being unable to fasten my seatbelt on a commercial airplane full of passengers. Note to flight attendants; an ounce of discretion would have been appreciated a ton. At the end of a dream gondola ride in Venice, I was unable to hoist my heft out of the gondola. When a very kind fellow passenger attempted to help me, he came within an eyelash of ending up in the Grand Canal.

I've tried pills, potions, lotions, "plans," "systems," "breakthroughs" and "revolutions." I have faithfully followed diets consisting of 1 hard boiled egg and 3 prunes for breakfast, a half cup of cottage cheese and 3 rye crackers for lunch, a lamb chop and a half cup each of green beans and beets for dinner with all the black coffee, diet soda and water that I wanted. I drank shakes, combined foods, counted percentages of carbs to proteins to fats, eliminated entire food groups from my diet and I've eaten prepared calorie controlled meals consisting of ..... actually, I don't know what they consisted of.

I have purchased shoes, tights, leotards, sweats, machines, gizmos, gadgets, memberships and "I went for the burn." I've been tested, counseled and advised. The only solution I stopped short of is surgery. I believe God already engineered our bodies for optimum performance. We just don't listen to what our bodies tell us to do.

Eight years ago, my doctor discovered several very large nodules on my thyroid. "Nodules" are just another word for tumors. Instead of being worried about cancer, my first thought was "Whoopee! I'll take a pill every day and be thin!" WRONG! Within 3 years following thyroid removal surgery my heft exploded to 301 pounds. After extensive research about the thyroid I discovered it is **more** difficult to lose or control weight after a complete thyroid removal.

A short while later during an annual check-up, my doctor did an EKG. She saw something suspicious and ordered a stress test. The results of the stress test indicated the possibility of a blocked artery. An angiogram was ordered. Thankfully, the angiogram showed perfectly clear arteries.

However, it was devastating to see the scale register 301 pounds and to experience the possibility of artery blockage at age 51. However, I believe I finally heard what my body had been telling me all my life; just take care of me and strive to be healthy. I also realized that nothing I had done in the past was going to help me to take care of my body or to be healthy.

I reviewed everything I had tried and asked myself why it hadn't worked for me. Five facts emerged that formed the foundation of a true breakthrough for me. The Five Facts helped me to lose 165 pounds and to maintain the weight loss for 3 years as of the date of this writing.

I am not suggesting that you follow my program exactly. Instead, use my program as a guide to develop a program that is comfortable for you and fits your life.

I do suggest, however, that you consult with your doctor before beginning your program. Your health is the first concern and your doctor will tell you if you are able to follow this eating and activity program.

In this book, I share with you

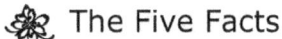 The Five Facts.

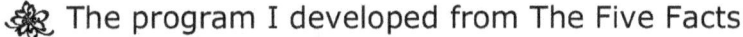 The program I developed from The Five Facts.

Healthy, delicious recipes I created to compliment the program.

The Five Facts

Fact 1

There is no better authority about what is best for our bodies than our own bodies. Why else would we feel so good when we do the right things and so bad when we do the wrong things?

So, listen to your body first. If you are exercising and it hurts, stop. If you are hungry, eat something. If you are full, stop eating.

Fact 2

Eliminating an entire food group from your diet, even temporarily, is not healthy, will not help you to lose weight or to maintain a weight loss. The process of eliminating a food group only to replace the missing nutrients with a complicated combination of other foods or supplements has always baffled me. If the elimination is not medically required, your body will thank you for the real thing.

I consider dessert a food group so I include desserts in this fact. Your goal is to include some of each food group in your diet to provide variety and the complete vitamins and minerals your body needs to maintain and fuel itself. Desserts provide fuel for your soul so they are absolutely necessary!

Fact 3

It's all about the old-fashioned calorie, period. However, I learned 2 very important facts about calories. First, it is the total number of calories consumed per **week** not per day that is important. It is an unrealistic goal to try and eat the same number of calories each and every day. Second, it is an equally unrealistic goal to maintain good health consuming less than 1000 calories per day.

Fact 4

Moderate exercise works hand-in-hand with the old-fashioned calorie. I stress the word moderate because if the exercise hurts or is too strenuous for your body, you will get frustrated with it. Choose an activity you enjoy rather than the latest fad exercise. Most importantly, **don't** go for the burn.

Fact 5

***If you can't do it for the rest of your life,
it won't work.***

My Program

Fact 3, "It's all about the old-fashioned calorie, period" is the foundation of the program I developed for myself. To determine your proper weekly calorie goal, refer to the web site www.caloriecontrol.org. Scroll down to "Healthy Weight Tool Kit." Click on "Diet Assessment." Fill in your gender, height, current weight and activity level. Click "re-assess my goal." Your healthy weight range, BMI and the daily number of calories you require to maintain your current weight or lose weight will be provided. Multiply your daily number of calories by 7 for your weekly calorie goal.

If you don't have Internet access, you and your trusty calculator can determine your weekly calorie goal. Multiply your current weight by 10 calories. If you do at least 30 minutes of exercise 3 times per week, multiply your current weight by an additional 3 calories. Add the results together to determine your proper daily calorie goal. To safely lose approximately 2 pounds per week, subtract 500 calories from that total and multiply the balance by 7 for your weekly calorie goal.

I spend a few minutes each evening to plan my menu for the next day. Fact 2, "Eliminating an entire food group from your diet is not healthy" is my guide in menu planning. I include foods from each food group and build a menu of meals with tasty variety that cumulatively stay within my weekly calorie goal.

It works for me to consider 1 day a week as a special food day. It may or may not involve a holiday or a special occasion. Nevertheless, it is the day I plan to eat certain special foods otherwise known as the Dessert Food Group.

I do not consider it a cheat day because the calories for all of my special foods are included in my weekly calorie goal. Therefore, I savor every one of the special foods I plan for with complete enjoyment and no guilt.

For the activity portion of my program, I follow Fact 4, "Moderate exercise works hand in hand with the old-fashioned calorie." I have always enjoyed bicycling and the Hula Hoop. When I began I exercised for 5 minutes on the stationery bike followed by 5 minutes with the Hula Hoop. It doesn't sound as though 5 minutes of each activity would be very effective, right? But, believe me, at 301 pounds, it was as effective for me as a 60 minute jog for a 150 pound person. Bending over to pick up the Hula Hoop 35 times in 5 minutes was effective enough! However, because I enjoy the activities and they didn't hurt I continued and gradually increased the time as I was able to.

Because I am eating a variety of normal food, including foods from the Dessert Food Group, and doing activities that I enjoy my program has evolved into my lifestyle. At present, almost 4 years after I began I continue to "live the program" and am maintaining the weight loss that I achieved.

I have seen television commercials for weight loss products that imply after you lose the desired weight you can eat whatever you want. I have not found this to be entirely true. After I reached the weight I wanted to maintain, I did learn 2 more facts . I call them The Bittersweet Facts.

Maintenance

The Bittersweet Facts

Fact 1

As our bodies shed excess pounds, they require fewer calories. Therefore, periodically recheck your weekly calorie goal. After you reach your goal weight, trial and error is the best method to determine the proper weekly calorie goal to maintain your weight loss. We all know that consuming too many calories results in weight gain, but I learned that consuming too few calories will produce the same result.

During the time it took you to achieve your desired weight, you learned portion sizes. This knowledge will serve you well to maintain your desired weight. You will be able to eat anything you want because you now know that a serving of *any* food is not the size of the Thanksgiving Day turkey platter.

Fact 2

Because our bodies are so wonderfully adaptive, it is necessary to keep them guessing. Otherwise, believe it or not, your chosen activity will become too easy. So, as you progress, gradually increase your time or the number of repetitions you perform. I keep my body guessing by adding new activities and alternating my workouts week to week.

Along the way I have added arm exercises using 15 pound weights, crunches while sitting on a balance ball, jump roping and a dance routine based on the Sicilian folk dance, the Tarantella. The variety of activities keep the workouts interesting and keep my body guessing.

<u>Routine 1</u>
stationery bike - 20 minutes
arm weights - 10 minutes
Tarantella - 10 minutes
crunches - 100 repetitions
Hula Hoop - 5 minutes
stretching - 5 minutes

<u>Routine 2</u>
stationery bike - 15 minutes
arm weights - 10 minutes
crunches - 100 repetitions
stationery bike - 15 minutes
Hula Hoop - 5 minutes
stretching - 5 minutes

<u>Routine 3</u>
stationery bike - 15 minutes
arm weights - 10 minutes
crunches - 100 repetitions
Hula Hoop & jump rope - alternate 5 minutes each
for a total of 15 minutes
stretching - 5 minutes

Whatever you choose to do to keep your body guessing, remember Fact 4 .... **moderation.**

The Recipes

I created this collection of recipes to compliment the menu planning portion of my program. Some of the recipes were inspired by family favorites, some from traditional Italian recipes and others are the result of a dream followed by many kitchen experiments.

Regardless of the inspiration, readily available ingredients and ease of preparation are important to me when I cook. Therefore, I use only those ingredients that are commonly found at just about any grocery store and prepare them simply. I believe my Italian genes show themselves in these recipes. The most important rules in Italian cooking are to use the freshest ingredients possible and then to do as little as possible to them in the preparation.
I prefer to enjoy the flavors of the ingredients themselves, so you will notice I don't use an abundance of spices and seasonings. Feel free to adjust these recipes to your taste preference.

Since I learned that it's all about the old-fashioned calorie, I have only included the calorie count per serving. By using a variety of fresh, whole ingredients that were created by God, limiting ingredients that were created by man and preparing the dishes with cooking methods such as roasting, braising in broths, steaming and grilling without fats, I am comfortable that all the remaining nutritional values are well within suggested healthy amounts. When the ingredients in a recipe call for "1 recipe ...." the calories for the second recipe are included in the calorie count for the main recipe.

Breakfast

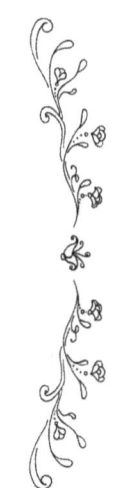
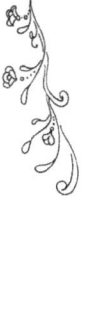

Cereal Parfait
Hot Cereal Parfait
Sicilian Cereal Parfait
Sicilian Breakfast Polenta
Breakfast Sandwich 1
Breakfast Sandwich 2
Scrambler Souffle
Stuffed French Toast
Cranberry Orange Almond Syrup
Roasted "Nutty" Grapefruit
Fruit and Cheese Breakfast Bowl
Roasted Fruit Two Ways
Yogurt Parfait
Biscuits
Breakfast Fruit Shortcake
Breakfast Bread
Apple Butter

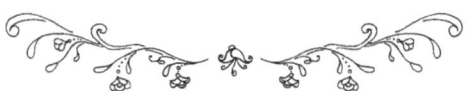

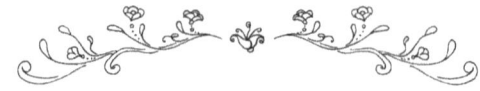

Cereal Parfait
2 servings - 309 calories each

2 cups	whole grain cereal
12 ounces	fat-free yogurt (any flavor)
4	dried apricots, chopped or 1/2 cup raisins
2 Tbsp	chopped walnuts

Layer the ingredients into each of 2 cereal bowls in the quantities following;

1/2 cup cereal
3 ounces yogurt
1 chopped apricot or 1/8 cup raisins
1/2 cup cereal
3 ounces yogurt
1 chopped apricot or 1/8 cup raisins
1 Tbsp walnuts

ENJOY!

Hot Cereal Parfait
1 serving - 349 calories

3 Tbsp	Farina Hot Cereal
3/4 cup	water
1	ripe peach, pear or banana, sliced
8 tsp	fat-free vanilla yogurt
1 Tbsp	chopped walnuts

Combine Farina and water in a microwave-safe bowl with a vented lid. Microwave, covered, on high for 1 minute. Stir and let sit for 1 minute. Microwave, covered, for 30 seconds more or until the cereal is to your desired consistency.

Spoon half of the Farina into a serving bowl. Arrange half of fruit on top of Farina followed by 4 tsp of yogurt, the remaining Farina, the remaining fruit and the remaining 4 tsp of yogurt. Top with the walnuts.

ENJOY!

Sicilian Cereal Parfait
<u>1 serving - 306 calories</u>

1 cup	crispy, whole grain cereal
2 Tbsp	freshly brewed coffee
1/4 cup	raisins
1/2	Ricotta Dip 2 recipe (see Dressings, Relishes and Spreads)

Pour cereal into a serving bowl. Sprinkle coffee over the cereal. Top with raisins. Spoon Ricotta Dip over top.

* The inspiration for this recipe came from a visit to Italy. While there, I noticed the Italians do not pour milk over their cereal. Instead, they spoon their coffee over it. I tried it, love it and have never gone back to milk!

ENJOY!

Sicilian Breakfast Polenta
2 servings - 350 calories each

4 slices	deli smoked ham, diced
1/2 cup	fat-free ricotta cheese
2 cups	fresh spinach, torn into small pieces
pinch	nutmeg
1/4 tsp	ground black pepper
1/4 cup	raisins
1/2	2.2 lb. tube prepared polenta

In a medium size bowl, combine the ham, ricotta, spinach, nutmeg, pepper and raisins. Mix well.

Divide the polenta into 6 equal slices. Place the slices in a single layer on a microwave-safe dish. Top each with 1/6 of the ricotta mixture. Cover the dish with microwave-safe plastic wrap and vent it. Microwave on high 5 minutes until heated through.

ENJOY!

Breakfast Sandwich 1
2 servings - 233 calories each

6 slices	Canadian bacon
1	large tomato, cut into 6 slices
2 Tbsp	grated Parmigiano Reggiano cheese
2 tsp	dried oregano
4 slices	whole wheat bread

Preheat oven to 350 degrees.

On a large baking sheet, lay the Canadian bacon and tomato slices in a single layer. Sprinkle the cheese and oregano evenly on the tomato slices. Bake for 5 minutes or until the cheese is golden brown.

Make 2 sandwiches by arranging 3 slices of bacon topped with 3 tomato slices between 2 slices of bread.

ENJOY!

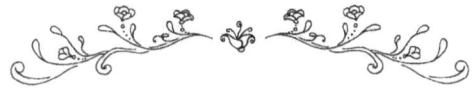

Breakfast Sandwich 2
2 servings - 435 calories each

2 Tbsp	light mayonnaise
4 slices	whole wheat bread
4 slices	deli smoked ham
1	medium apple, cored and thinly sliced
2 slices	2% milk American cheese
2 Tbsp	Dijon mustard

Spray a large skillet with non-stick cooking spray. Spread 1 Tbsp of mayonnaise on each of 2 slices of bread. Layer each bread with 2 slices of ham, 1/2 of the apple slices and 1 slice of cheese. Spread 1 Tbsp of mustard on the remaining 2 slices of bread and set 1 on each sandwich.

Heat the skillet on medium-high heat and cook the sandwiches to a golden brown. Remove the sandwiches to a plate and spray the skillet again with non-stick cooking spray. Cook the other side of the sandwiches to a golden brown.

ENJOY!

Scrambler Souffle
2 servings - 324 calories each

1 cup	potato gnocchi, uncooked *
3 ounces	deli smoked ham, diced
1	tomato, cored and chopped
2 cups	fresh spinach, chopped
1 cup	egg substitute
1/8 tsp	salt
1/8 tsp	ground black pepper
2 Tbsp	grated Parmigiano Reggiano

* potato gnocchi can be found either in the pasta aisle or amongst the Italian food in the ethnic food aisle.

Preheat oven to 425 degrees.

Spray 2 10- ounce oven-safe ramekin bowls with butter flavored non-stick cooking spray. Layer each ramekin with half of the gnocchi, ham, tomato and spinach. Pour 1/2 cup of the egg substitute over each. Sprinkle each with half of the salt, pepper and cheese.

Coat one side of a piece of aluminum foil large enough to cover the ramekins with non-stick cooking spray. Cover the ramekins with the foil and bake for 25 minutes. Let sit 5 minutes before serving.

ENJOY!

Stuffed French Toast with Syrup
2 servings - 568 calories each

2 cups	orange juice
1/4 cup	dried cranberries
1/4 cup	fat-free ricotta cheese
1 Tbsp	honey
4 slices	country style Italian bread
3/4 cup	egg substitute
2 Tbsp	chopped almonds

Combine orange juice and cranberries in a small sauce pot. Bring to a boil over high heat. Reduce heat and simmer 15 to 20 minutes, stirring occasionally, until thickened to a syrup consistency.

Meanwhile, in a small bowl, combine ricotta and honey and mix well.

Spray a large skillet with butter flavored non-stick cooking spray. Divide the ricotta mixture evenly between 2 slices of bread. Top each with one of the remaining slices of bread. Place the egg substitute in a bowl large enough to dip the French toasts in. Set the skillet over medium-high heat. Dip each sandwich in the egg substitute coating both sides well. Set in skillet and cook until golden brown on both sides.

Add the almonds to the thickened syrup and stir well.

ENJOY!

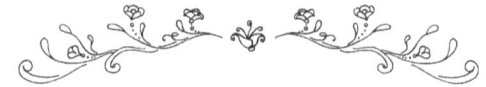

Roasted "Nutty" Grapefruit
2 servings - 123 calories each

1	grapefruit, peeled and sectioned
1-1/2 Tbsp	honey
2 Tbsp	shredded coconut

Preheat oven to 325 degrees. Spray a baking pan with non-stick cooking spray.

Place grapefruit sections in the prepared pan. Drizzle the honey evenly over the fruit. Sprinkle the coconut evenly on top.

Roast for 5 minutes or until the coconut is lightly toasted.

ENJOY!

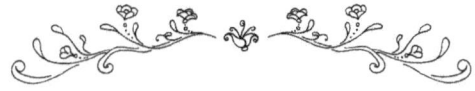

Fruit and Cheese Breakfast Bowl
2 servings - 346 calories each

14	strawberries, hulled and chopped
1	banana, chopped
1	pear , cored and chopped
1/2 tsp	ground ginger
2 cups	fat-free cottage cheese
2 Tbsp	pecans, chopped

In a medium size bowl, combine the strawberries, banana, pear and ginger. Stir together gently.

Place 1 cup of cottage cheese in each serving bowl. Top each with half of the fruit mixture. Sprinkle each with 1 Tbsp of pecans.

ENJOY!

Roasted Fruit Two Ways
4 servings

First Way - 146 calories each

1	grapefruit, peeled and segmented
1	orange, peeled and segmented
1	peach, pitted and sliced
1 cup	strawberries, hulled and sliced
3 Tbsp	pine nuts
2 Tbsp	hot water
4 tsp	honey
1/2 tsp	vanilla extract

Second Way - 152 calories each

1	pear, cored and sliced
1	apple, cored and sliced
1 cup	red grapes
2	plums, pitted and sliced
3 Tbsp	chopped walnuts
2 Tbsp	hot water
4 tsp	honey
1/2 tsp	vanilla extract
1 tsp	lemon juice

Preheat oven to 375 degrees.

In an 8 x 8 square casserole, combine the fruit and nuts.

In a small bowl, whisk together the remaining ingredients.

Pour the syrup over the fruit and nuts and stir to coat. Bake 15 minutes, stirring halfway through the cooking time.

ENJOY!

Yogurt Parfait
2 servings - 217 calories each

1/2 cup	whole grain cereal
1 Tbsp	chopped pecans or walnuts
12 ounces	fat-free vanilla yogurt
1	banana, diced or 1 pear, cored and diced
8	strawberries, cored and sliced

Place the cereal in a plastic bag and tie the bag closed. With a glass or rolling pin, gently crush the cereal. Be careful not to crush it into a powder. Add the pecans and shake the bag to evenly distribute the pecans with the cereal. Set aside.

Use 2-cup clear, glass mugs or parfait glasses. In each glass, make 2 layers of the ingredients in the quantities following;

3 ounces yogurt
1/4 of the banana or pear
1/4 of the strawberries
1/4 of the cereal mixture

ENJOY!

Biscuits
7 servings - 161 calories each

1 cup	all-purpose flour
1 cup	whole wheat flour
2 tsp	baking powder
1/2 tsp	baking soda
1/4 tsp	salt
1/2 cup	cold, fat-free cream cheese, diced
1 cup	fat-free vanilla yogurt
1 tsp	honey

Preheat oven to 375 degrees. Spray a baking sheet with non-stick cooking spray. Set aside.

In a large mixing bowl, combine the flours, baking powder, baking soda and salt. Briskly whisk the dry ingredients together. Add the cream cheese and, with your fingers, blend the cream cheese into the flour until the mixture looks like coarse crumbs. Set aside.

In a small bowl, stir together the yogurt and honey. Add to the flour mixture and gently toss with a fork to moisten the flour. If necessary, add ice cold water a Tbsp at a time until the dough comes together completely. Knead the dough in the bowl a few times.

Drop 1/3 cupfuls of dough onto baking sheet. Leave approximately 2 inches of space all around each biscuit. Bake 10 to 12 minutes until golden brown. Refrigerate any leftovers.

ENJOY!

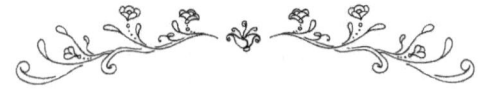

Breakfast Fruit Shortcake
2 servings - 272 calories each

2	ripe peaches, pitted and coarsely chopped
1 tsp	vanilla extract
1/8 tsp	ginger
1/4 tsp	dried basil
2	biscuits (see preceding Biscuits recipe)
4 Tbsp	fat-free vanilla yogurt

In a medium bowl, combine peaches, vanilla, ginger and basil. Mix well.

Set 1 biscuit on each serving dish. Spoon the peaches over biscuits, dividing the peach mixture evenly between the two servings. Top each serving with 2 Tbsp of yogurt.

Nectarines, plums, blueberries or strawberries can be substituted for the peaches.

ENJOY!

Breakfast Bread
10 slices - 177 calories each

1 cup	all-purpose flour
1/2 cup	whole wheat flour
1/2 cup	quick cooking oatmeal
1/8 tsp	salt
2 tsp	baking powder
3/4 tsp	baking soda
3/4 tsp	ground cinnamon
1/3 cup	honey
1-1/4 cup	unsweetened chunky applesauce
1	large egg
2 tsp	vanilla extract
1/3 cup	chopped walnuts
5	walnut halves
1 Tbsp	quick cooking oatmeal

Preheat oven to 325 degrees.

Coat an 8 x 4 loaf pan with non-stick cooking spray. Set aside.

In a large bowl, combine the flours, 1/2 cup oatmeal, salt, baking powder, baking soda and cinnamon. Whisk together well.

In a separate bowl, combine the honey, applesauce, egg and vanilla. Whisk together well.

Add the applesauce mixture to the flour mixture and stir just to moisten the dry ingredients. Fold in the chopped walnuts. Spoon the batter into the prepared loaf pan, smoothing the top of the loaf. Tap the pan on the counter a few times to evenly distribute the batter.

Breakfast Bread
continued

Make a slash long ways through the center of the loaf. Lay the walnut halves in the slash and sprinkle the 1 Tbsp of oatmeal on top.

Bake 50 to 55 minutes until a toothpick inserted in the center comes out clean. If the top browns too quickly, cover loosely with aluminum foil.

Cool in pan 15 minutes. Remove from pan and let cool completely on a wire rack.

ENJOY!

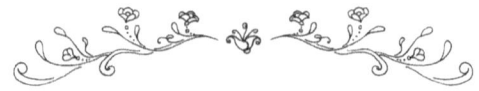

Apple Butter
40 Tbsp - 12 calories each

4 pounds	medium apples (approx. 5), cored, peeled and sliced
1/3 cup	apple juice
1/4 tsp	salt
1 tsp	ground cinnamon
1/2 tsp	ground nutmeg
1/8 tsp	allspice
2 tsp	vanilla extract
1 Tbsp	lemon juice

Place all ingredients in a large pot. Stir well to distribute seasoning evenly. Cover and bring to a simmer over medium heat. Cook 15 to 25 minutes, stirring occasionally. When apples are very tender, transfer to a food processor bowl. Pulse in short spurts. The butter should be smooth, but thick. Be careful not to over process.

The butter will remain fresh, refrigerated for 2 weeks.

ENJOY!

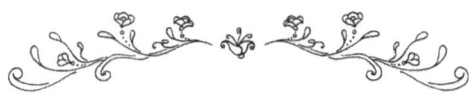

Dressings, Relishes, Spreads

Quick Creamy Italian Dressing
Fresh Cranberry Relish 1
Fresh Cranberry Relish 2
Ricotta Dip 1
Ricotta Dip 2
Ricotta Dip 3
Eggplant and Artichoke Spread
Red Pepper and Tomato Spread

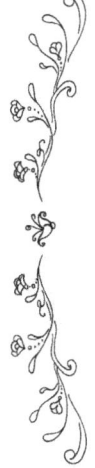
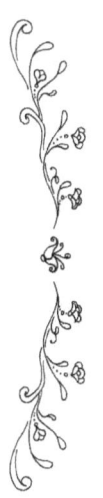
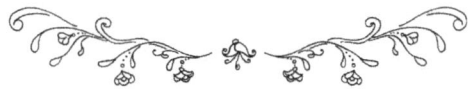

Quick Creamy Italian Dressing
2 servings - 33 calories each

2 Tbsp	fat-free sour cream
6 Tbsp	bottled fat-free Italian dressing

Whisk sour cream and Italian dressing together until smooth. Pour over salad.

ENJOY!

Fresh Cranberry Relish 1
16 Tbsp - 10 calories each

1 Tbsp	pecan halves
1/2 cup	fresh cranberries, rinsed and drained
1/2 cup	pineapple cubes in juice
1/8 tsp	salt

Combine all ingredients in bowl of food processor. Pulse in short spurts. The finished relish should have distinguishable pieces of pecans, cranberries and pineapple.

Serve the relish alongside turkey, chicken or pork. It is also great as a spread for sandwiches or a topping for bruschetta.

ENJOY!

Fresh Cranberry Relish 2
16 Tbsp - 13 calories each

1 Tbsp	pecan halves
1/2 cup	fresh cranberries, rinsed and drained
1/2	medium pear
1/2	medium apple
2 Tbsp	fat-free vanilla yogurt
1/8 tsp	salt

Combine all ingredients in bowl of food processor. Pulse in short spurts. The finished relish should have distinguishable pieces of pecans, cranberries, pear and apple.

This relish is also great to top toast, oatmeal or ice cream and as a dip for fresh fruit, cookies or biscotti.

ENJOY!

Ricotta Dip 1
2 servings - 72 calories each

1/2 cup	fat-free ricotta cheese
1/8 tsp	salt
1-1/2 tsp	honey
1 tsp	vanilla extract
1 tsp	mini semi-sweet chocolate chips

In a medium bowl combine ricotta, salt, honey and vanilla. Mix well. Gently fold in the chocolate chips.

Serve as a dip for fresh fruit and biscotti, layered in a fresh fruit parfait or as a topping for cereal, oatmeal or toast.

ENJOY!

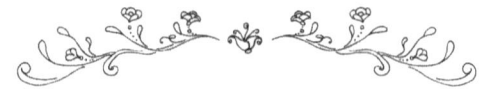
Ricotta Dip 2
2 servings - 86 calories each

1 tsp	instant coffee
1 tsp	warm water
3/4 cup	fat-free ricotta cheese
1/8 tsp	salt
1-3/4 tsp	honey
1 tsp	vanilla extract

Place instant coffee and water in a medium size bowl. Stir well to dissolve coffee. Add ricotta, salt, honey and vanilla. Stir to combine well. Refrigerate until ready to use.

ENJOY!

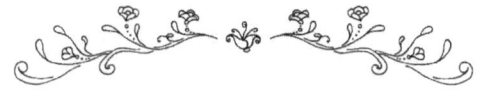

Ricotta Dip 3
<u>16 Tbsp - 10 calories each</u>

1 cup	fat-free ricotta cheese
1/4 tsp	granulated garlic
1/4 tsp	salt
1/4 tsp	ground black pepper
1/2 tsp	dried oregano

In a medium size bowl, combine all ingredients and mix well.

Serve as a dip for fresh vegetables or as a spread for sandwiches.

ENJOY!

Eggplant and Artichoke Spread
4 servings - 49 calories each

1/2	medium eggplant, peeled and cubed
6	artichoke hearts in water
1/4 tsp	salt
1/4 tsp	ground black pepper
1/2 tsp	dried oregano
1/2 tsp	dried basil
1/8 tsp	granulated garlic
1/8 tsp	crushed red pepper flakes
1 Tbsp	grated Romano cheese

Place the eggplant and artichoke hearts in a large microwave-safe bowl. Add approximately 2 inches of water. Microwave on high 10 minutes. Strain the mixture well to drain the remaining water. Return the mixture to the bowl.

With the back of a fork, mash the vegetables well. Add the remaining ingredients and mix well. Refrigerate until serving time.

In addition to being a delicious sandwich spread, this is a wonderful dip for raw vegetables. Serve it as a relish alongside fish. It is also perfect as an appetizer set atop whole grain crackers or toasted bread.

ENJOY!

Red Pepper and Tomato Spread
4 servings - 47 calories each

2	red peppers, stemmed, seeded and chopped
6	plum tomatoes, cored, seeded and cubed
1/4 tsp	salt
1/4 tsp	ground black pepper
1/4 tsp	crushed red pepper flakes
1/2 tsp	dried oregano
1/2 tsp	dried basil
1/8 tsp	granulated garlic
1 Tbsp + 1 tsp	white balsamic vinegar
1/2 tsp	honey

Place the peppers and tomatoes in a large microwave-safe bowl. Add approximately 2 inches of water. Microwave on high 15 minutes. Strain the mixture well to drain the remaining water. Return the mixture to the bowl.

With the back of a fork, mash the vegetables well. Add the remaining ingredients and mix well. Refrigerate until serving time.

In addition to being delicious on sandwiches, this spread can also be used as a relish served with meats. Or, use it as an appetizer atop whole grain crackers and toasted bread with a sprinkle of grated Parmigiano.

ENJOY!

Appetizers, Snacks

Bruschetta
Eggplant Bruschetta 1
Eggplant Bruschetta 2
Eggplant Bruschetta 3
Italian Nachos
Italian Nachos Dippers
Roasted Squash Seeds

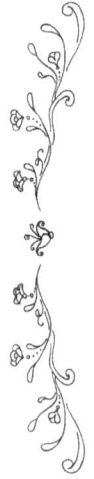

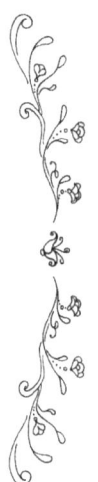

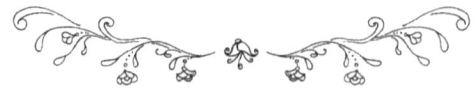

Bruschetta
2 servings - 140 calories each

1 Tbsp	extra-virgin olive oil
1 Tbsp	grated Romano cheese
1/8 tsp	ground black pepper
3	plum tomatoes, chopped
6	dried Sicilian black olives, chopped

* dried Sicilian black olives are available in the deli department of larger grocery stores or Italian markets. If you can't find them, substitute Gaeta or other black olive.

Into a medium size bowl, place olive oil, cheese, pepper, tomatoes and olives. Mix well.

Serve on Italian bread or crackers. (Not included in the calorie count.)

ENJOY!

Eggplant Bruschetta 1
4 servings - 106 calories each

1	large red, orange or yellow bell pepper
1	medium eggplant
1 Tbsp	extra-virgin olive oil
1/4 tsp	salt
1/4 tsp	ground black pepper
2 ounces	soft goat cheese

Remove the stem, core and seeds from the pepper and cut the pepper in half. Cut each half into 4 pieces. Remove the stem and peel from the eggplant and cut it into 8 - 1 inch thick slices.

Preheat the broiler.

Spray the outside of peppers and both sides of eggplant slices with butter flavored non-stick cooking spray. Arrange peppers and eggplant in a single layer on a baking sheet. Lightly brush each vegetable with the olive oil. Broil 15-20 minutes, turning them over halfway through the cooking time, until tender and browned.

Sprinkle eggplant with salt and pepper. Spread the goat cheese on the eggplant, dividing it equally between the eight slices. Top each with a slice of pepper.

ENJOY!

Eggplant Bruschetta 2
4 servings - 64 calories each

1	medium eggplant
8 tsp	prepared pesto sauce
8	cherry tomatoes, cut in half

Remove the stem and peel from the eggplant. Cut the eggplant into 8 - 1 inch thick slices. Spray both sides of eggplant with butter flavored non-stick cooking spray and arrange slices in a single layer on a baking sheet.

Preheat broiler.

Broil 15 to 20 minutes, turning the eggplant over halfway through the cooking time, until the eggplant is tender and golden brown.

Spread 1 tsp of pesto sauce on each eggplant slice. Top each with 2 cherry tomato halves.

ENJOY!

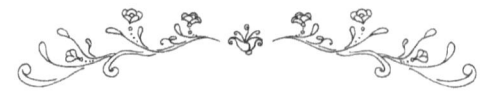

Eggplant Bruschetta 3
4 servings - 94 calories each

1	medium eggplant
2 ounces	gorgonzola cheese
8	walnut halves

Remove the stem and peel from the eggplant. Cut the eggplant into 8 - 1 inch thick slices. Spray both sides of eggplant with butter flavored non-stick cooking spray and arrange slices in a single layer on a baking sheet.

Preheat broiler.

Broil 15 to 20 minutes, turning the eggplant over halfway through the cooking time, until the eggplant is tender and golden brown.

Spread approximately 1/4 ounce of gorgonzola on each eggplant slice. Top each with a walnut half.

ENJOY!

Italian Nachos
<u>15 servings - 319 calories each</u>

1 pound	bulk Italian sausage
1/2	medium red onion, cut into 1 inch slices
1/2	stick pepperoni, diced
1 14 ounce	can crushed tomatoes
2 tsp	dried oregano
1/2 tsp	ground black pepper
1-1/2 cup	part skim ricotta cheese
1/2 cup	fresh basil, torn
1/2 tsp	granulated garlic
pinch	salt
1 2.25 ounce	can sliced black olives
1/2 cup	grated Romano cheese
1	recipe Italian Nachos Dippers (following recipe)

In a large skillet, saute sausage and onion until sausage is no longer pink and onion is translucent. Add pepperoni, crushed tomatoes, oregano and black pepper. Stir and simmer gently 10 minutes.

Meanwhile, in a medium bowl combine ricotta, basil, granulated garlic and salt. Mix well.

Spread ricotta mixture on a 7-1/2 x 10-1/2 serving dish. Top with sausage mixture. Add the black olives and sprinkle with the Romano cheese.

ENJOY!

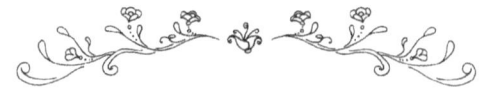

Italian Nachos Dippers
15 servings - 135 calories each

1 pound	pizza dough
1	medium zucchini, sliced into 30 discs
3	red, yellow or orange peppers, stems removed and sliced into a total of 30 strips.

Preheat oven to 400 degrees. Spray a baking sheet with non-stick cooking spray. Set aside.

Roll out the pizza dough into a large rectangle approximately 9 x 12. Cut the dough into 30 strips approximately 1-1/4 x 3. Lay the strips in a single layer on the baking sheet. Bake for 7 to 8 minutes or until golden brown and crispy.

Use crispy dippers, zucchini and peppers to scoop up the Italian Nachos.

ENJOY!

Roasted Squash Seeds
1 ounce (approx. 85 seeds) - 127 calories
(recipe yield will vary)

	the seeds from 1 fresh pumpkin, butternut squash or acorn squash
2 Tbsp	extra-virgin olive oil
1 tsp	salt

Clean pulp from seeds and set seeds aside to dry for at least 1 hour. Depending on how many seeds you have, you may need to roast them in more than 1 batch.

Place seeds in a bowl. Drizzle with olive oil and sprinkle with salt. Stir seeds well to coat.

Conventional Oven
Preheat oven to 325 degrees. Transfer seeds from bowl to a baking sheet and arrange them in a single layer. Roast for 15 to 25 minutes until seeds are golden brown and crunchy. Stir halfway through the cooking time.

Microwave Oven
Transfer seeds from bowl to a microwave-safe dish or pan and arrange them in a single layer. Microwave on high in 2 to 3 minute intervals until golden brown and crunchy.

ENJOY!

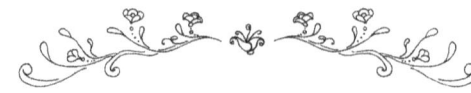

Salads

Tuna Salad
Sicilian Tuna Salad
Waldorf Salad with Chicken
Pasta Salad
A Different Panzanella Salad
Pear Waldorf Salad

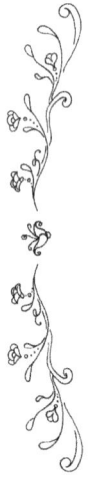
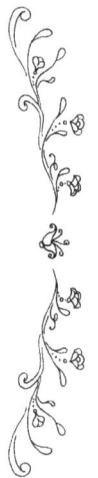
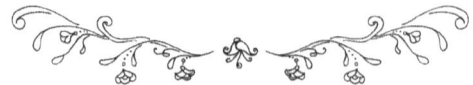

Tuna Salad
2 servings - 93 calories each

1	5 ounce can white albacore tuna in water
1 Tbsp	red onion, finely chopped
1/2	stalk celery, finely chopped
dash	ground black pepper
1 Tbsp	light mayonnaise
1 Tbsp	fat-free sour cream
1/2 tsp	prepared mustard
1/16 tsp	lemon juice
1/4 tsp	dried parsley

Drain tuna and place in a medium size bowl. Add onion, celery and pepper. Set aside.

In a separate, medium size bowl combine mayonnaise, sour cream, mustard, lemon juice and parsley. Mix well.

Add tuna mixture to mayonnaise mixture and stir well to thoroughly combine the two together.

Refrigerate at least 1 hour before serving.

ENJOY!

Sicilian Tuna Salad
2 servings - 250 calories each

1	7 ounce can albacore tuna in water, drained
1/4 tsp	ground black pepper, divided
1/4 tsp	dried oregano
1	clove garlic, minced
1/8 tsp	salt
3 Tbsp	Marsala wine
1-1/2 tsp	Dijon mustard
1 Tbsp	extra-virgin olive oil
1/4 cup	raisins
1 Tbsp	almonds, chopped

Place tuna in a medium size bowl. Season with 1/8 tsp of pepper and the oregano. Set aside.

In a small bowl, whisk together the garlic, salt, remaining 1/8 tsp pepper, Marsala, mustard and olive oil.

To the tuna, add the raisins and almonds. Mix well. Pour the dressing over the tuna mixture and mix well.

Refrigerate at least 1 hour before serving.

ENJOY!

Waldorf Salad with Chicken
4 servings - 310 calories each

1/3 cup	reduced fat mayonnaise
1/3 cup	fat-free sour cream
1 tsp	dried, crushed rosemary
1 Tbsp	lemon juice
1 Tbsp	honey
2 cups	cooked chicken, cubed
2	medium apples, coarsely chopped
1/4 cup	celery, thinly sliced
1/4 cup	dried apricots, chopped
1/3 cup	chopped walnuts

In a medium size bowl, whisk together the mayonnaise, sour cream, rosemary, lemon juice and honey. Add the chicken, apples, celery, apricots and walnuts. Mix together well. Cover and refrigerate at least 1 hour before serving.

Turkey and dried cranberries can be substituted for the chicken and apricots.

ENJOY!

Pasta Salad
12, 1/2 cup servings - 229 calories each

1 pound	dried mostaccioli or penne pasta
2 Tbsp	red wine vinegar
1/2 tsp	salt
1/4 tsp	ground black pepper
1/2 tsp	honey
1/2 tsp	dry mustard
1-1/2 tsp	dried basil
1/8 tsp	granulated garlic
1/3 cup	extra-virgin olive oil
3 ounces	hard salami, diced
1/4 cup	red onion, minced
1 can	2-1/4 ounces sliced black olives, drained
2 strips	roasted red peppers, coarsely chopped

Cook pasta according to package directions until very al dente. (The pasta will "cook" more in the dressing.) Rinse under cold running water and drain well.

In a large bowl, combine vinegar, salt, pepper, honey, mustard, basil and garlic. Whisk in olive oil. When the pasta is completely drained and dry, transfer it to the bowl with the dressing.

Add the salami, red onion, olives and red peppers. Stir gently to distribute the dressing evenly.

ENJOY!

A Different Panzanella Salad
4 servings - 258 calories each

1	garlic clove
1/8 tsp	salt
1/8 tsp	ground black pepper
2 Tbsp	red wine vinegar
4 Tbsp	extra-virgin olive oil
4 slices	day old country style Italian bread, cubed
1	tomato, cored, seeded and chopped
1/2	seedless cucumber, peeled and chopped
1/4	of a red onion, thinly sliced
1 stalk	celery, thinly sliced
1/2	head Romaine lettuce, chopped
4	basil leaves, thinly sliced

Set the garlic clove on cutting board. Sprinkle the salt over the garlic. Using the side of a knife, mash the garlic to form a paste. Transfer the garlic paste to a small bowl. Add the pepper and red wine vinegar. Whisk in the olive oil. Set aside.

On a large serving dish or platter, layer half of the bread, tomato, cucumber, onion, celery and lettuce. Pour half of the dressing over the salad. Make a second layer with the remaining ingredients. Pour the remaining dressing over the salad. Distribute the basil evenly over the top.

Set aside at room temperature 30 minutes before serving.

ENJOY!

Pear Waldorf Salad
2 servings - 268 calories each

2 Tbsp	fat-free sour cream
1 Tbsp	reduced fat mayonnaise
1 tsp	lemon juice
1/8 tsp	salt
2	pears, cored and chopped
1 cup	seedless red grapes, halved
2 Tbsp	chopped walnuts
1 ounce	gorgonzola cheese

In a large bowl, combine sour cream, mayonnaise, lemon juice and salt. Add pears, grapes and walnuts. Stir gently to combine.

Divide salad evenly between 2 serving plates. Sprinkle each with 1/2 ounce of gorgonzola.

ENJOY!

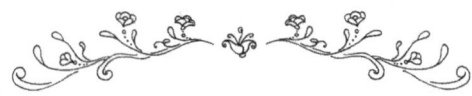

Sandwiches

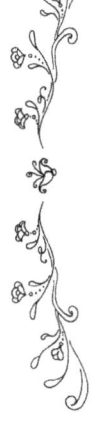

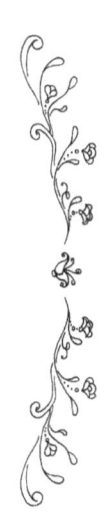

Citrus Tuna Sandwich
Turkey Salad with Walnuts Sandwich
Cheesy Turkey Melts
Chick'n Apple Salad Sandwich
Prosciutto, Provolone and Pear Sandwich
Grilled Steak Sandwich
Pear and Gorgonzola Sandwich
Not Your Kid's PB&J
Not Your Kid's PB&J, Either

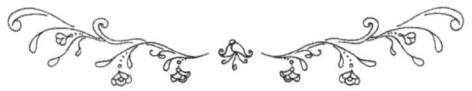

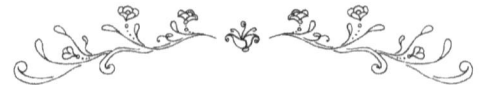

Citrus Tuna Sandwich
2 servings - 404 calories each

2 3 ounce	fresh tuna fillets
1/4 tsp	salt
1/4 tsp	ground black pepper
4 slices	whole wheat bread
2 tsp	extra-virgin olive oil
2 slices	provolone cheese
4	tissue thin slices of fresh orange

Season each tuna fillet with half of the salt and pepper. Spray a grill pan with non-stick cooking spray. Grill the fillets to your desired doneness. It is generally accepted for tuna fillets to be served red on the inside. However, I prefer them cooked through.

Drizzle 1 tsp olive oil on each of 2 slices of bread. Set 1 tuna fillet on each slice of bread. Lay 1 slice of cheese and 2 slices of orange on each tuna fillet. Top each with 1 of the remaining slices of bread.

ENJOY!

Turkey Salad with Walnuts Sandwich
2 servings - 313 calories each

2 Tbsp	light mayonnaise
1 Tbsp	fat-free sour cream
3/4 cup	cooked turkey breast, cubed
1/8 cup	celery, thinly sliced
2	dried apricots, chopped
1 Tbsp	chopped walnuts
1/8 tsp	salt
1/8 tsp	ground black pepper
2	romaine lettuce leaves
4 slices	whole wheat bread

In a medium size bowl, combine mayonnaise and sour cream. Add turkey, celery, apricots, walnuts, salt and pepper. Mix well. Refrigerate 30 minutes.

Make 2 sandwiches by using half of the turkey salad mixture and 1 lettuce leaf between 2 slices of bread.

ENJOY!

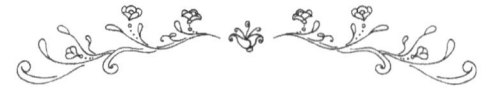

Cheesy Turkey Melts
2 servings - 320 calories each

1/2 cup	fat-free ricotta cheese
1/2 tsp	crushed rosemary
1/8 tsp	salt
4 slices	whole grain bread
4 ounces	sliced turkey breast
1	medium apple, cored and thinly sliced

Preheat oven to 375 degrees. Spray 2 pieces of aluminum foil large enough to wrap a sandwich, with non-stick cooking spray. Set aside.

In a small bowl, combine ricotta, rosemary and salt. Mix well. Spread the ricotta mixture on two slices of bread, dividing it evenly. Top each with half of the turkey, half of the apple slices and 1 of the remaining slices of bread.

Wrap each sandwich in 1 piece of the prepared foil, sealing the package tightly. Bake for 20 minutes or until the sandwiches are hot and bubbly.

ENJOY!

Chick'n Apple Salad Sandwich
2 servings - 322 calories each

3 Tbsp	plain, Greek yogurt
1-1/2 Tbsp	strawberry jam
3/4 cup	cooked chicken breast, cubed
1/2	medium apple, chopped
1 Tbsp	chopped walnuts
1/8 tsp	salt
1/8 tsp	ground black pepper
2	romaine lettuce leaves
4 slices	whole wheat bread

In a medium size bowl, combine yogurt and jam. Mix well. Add chicken, apple, walnuts, salt and pepper. Mix gently to combine all ingredients. Refrigerate 30 minutes.

Make 2 sandwiches by using half of the chicken salad mixture and 1 lettuce leaf between 2 slices of bread.

ENJOY!

Prosciutto, Provolone and Pear Sandwich
2 servings - 365 calories each

1-1/2 tsp	extra-virgin olive oil
1 Tbsp	red wine vinegar
1/8 tsp	ground black pepper
2 cups	fresh spinach
2 Tbsp	red onion, thinly slivered
4 slices	whole wheat bread
2 slices	thinly sliced prosciutto
2 slices	provolone cheese
1	ripe pear, cored and thinly sliced

In a medium size bowl, whisk together the olive oil, vinegar and pepper. Add the spinach and onion and toss to coat the vegetables with dressing.

Divide the spinach mixture evenly between two slices of bread. Top each with 1 slice of prosciutto, 1 slice of provolone, half of the pear slices and 1 of the remaining slices of bread.

ENJOY!

Grilled Steak Sandwich
2 servings - 394 calories each

2	2 ounce sandwich steaks
	salt and ground black pepper, to taste
4	small zucchini
1	large portobello mushroom
2	medium size submarine rolls
1	medium tomato, cored and thinly sliced
	dried basil, to taste
1 slice	red onion, thinly slivered

Season the sandwich steaks with salt and pepper to taste and set aside.

Cut stems off the zucchini and cut the zucchini longwise into 1/4 inch thick slices. Slice the portobello into 1/4 inch thick slices.

Spray a grill pan with non-stick cooking spray. Set the pan over medium-high heat. Lay the zucchini and portobello slices on the pan and grill 2 minutes on each side until tender and browned. Remove from pan onto a plate. Season with salt and pepper to taste. Cover and set aside to keep warm. Add the steaks to the pan and grill 1-1/2 minutes on each side. Sandwich steaks cook quickly. Be careful not to overcook because they will become tough.

Cut the rolls in half. Make sandwiches by layering a steak, 1/2 each of the zucchini, portobello, tomato and onion on each sub roll bottom. Sprinkle with basil and top with sub roll top.

ENJOY!

Pear and Gorgonzola Sandwich
2 sandwiches - 315 calories each

4 slices	whole grain bread
2 ounces	gorgonzola cheese
2 Tbsp	chopped walnuts
2 tsp	honey
1	pear, cored and thinly sliced

Crumble gorgonzola on 2 slices of bread, dividing it equally. Top each with 1 Tbsp of walnuts, 1 tsp of honey, half of the pear slices and 1 of the remaining slices of bread.

ENJOY!

Not Your Kid's PB&J
1 serving - 437 calories

2 slices	whole grain bread
1 Tbsp	peanut butter, creamy or chunky
2 ounces	smoked ham
1	fresh apricot, sliced
1	romaine lettuce leaf
1 tsp	honey

Spread the peanut butter on 1 slice of bread. Layer on the ham, sliced apricot and romaine leaf. Drizzle the honey on the remaining slice of bread. Set the bread with the honey toward the romaine, on the sandwich.

Turkey and a peach can be substituted for the ham and apricot.

ENJOY!

Not Your Kid's PB&J Either
2 servings - 325 calories each

4 slices	whole wheat bread
2 Tbsp	peanut butter, creamy or chunky
2 Tbsp	mini semi-sweet chocolate chips
1	peach, pitted and thinly sliced

Spread 1 Tbsp of peanut butter on each of 2 slices of bread. Sprinkle 1 Tbsp of chocolate chips on top of the peanut butter on each bread. Lay half of the peach slices on each. Top each with a slice of bread.

Spray a grill pan or skillet with butter flavored non-stick cooking spray and heat over medium-high heat. Gently brown the sandwiches on both sides, re-spraying the pan for the second side, if necessary.

ENJOY!

Soups and Stews

Tomato Quinoa Soup
Fresh Tomato Soup
Minestrone
Roasted Minestrone
Mom's Chicken Soup
Vegetable Meatballs
Beans 'n Greens Soup
Pasta e Fagioli
Vegetable Stew
Thanksgiving Chili
Italian Chili
Cabbage, Mushroom and Pork Soup
3 Days After the Pot Roast Soup

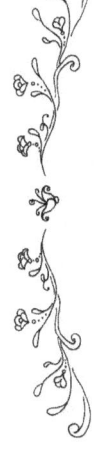
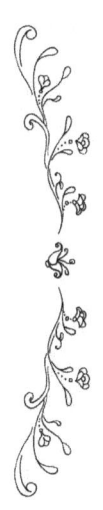
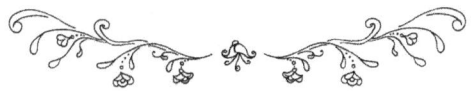

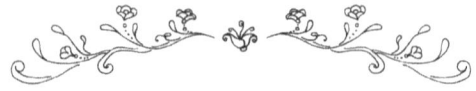

Tomato Quinoa Soup
12, 1 cup servings - 113 calories each

2 Tbsp	extra-virgin olive oil
1/4	medium red onion, chopped
1	stalk celery, chopped
4 slices	Canadian bacon, coarsely chopped
1 cup	quinoa, rinsed well
1	28 ounce can whole plum tomatoes
8 cups	chicken broth
1/2 tsp	salt
1/2 tsp	ground black pepper
1/2 tsp	dried basil
1/8 tsp	granulated garlic

In a medium size soup pot combine the olive oil, onion and celery. Saute until tender approximately 3 to 4 minutes. Add Canadian bacon and saute until browned. Add quinoa and toast for 2 minutes. Crush the tomatoes with your hands and add to pot along with 1 cup water. Stir well and simmer for 10 minutes. Add chicken broth, salt, pepper, basil and garlic. Cover and simmer 30 minutes, stirring occasionally, until quinoa is tender.

ENJOY!

Fresh Tomato Soup
14, 1 cup servings - 63 calories each

2 lbs. (4 large)	tomatoes, cored, seeded and cut in half
3 Tbsp	extra-virgin olive oil, divided
1 28 ounce	can plum tomatoes in juice
2	garlic cloves
1	stalk celery, chopped
1/4	medium red onion, chopped
6 cups	chicken broth
1 cup	tomato puree
1/2 tsp	salt
1/2 tsp	ground black pepper
1 tsp	dried basil
1	bay leaf

Preheat oven to 400 degrees.

Place tomatoes cut side down in roasting pan. Drizzle with 2 Tbsp olive oil. Roast 20 to 30 minutes until tender and slightly charred. Cool and remove skins.

Drain plum tomatoes reserving the juice. Place roasted tomatoes, plum tomatoes and garlic in food processor and puree.

In a medium size soup pot over medium-high heat, place remaining Tbsp of olive oil, celery and onion. Saute until tender. Add broth, tomato puree, the roasted tomato mixture, the reserved juice, salt, pepper, basil and bay leaf. Bring to a boil and simmer gently, uncovered, 20 to 30 minutes. Remove bay leaf before serving.

ENJOY!

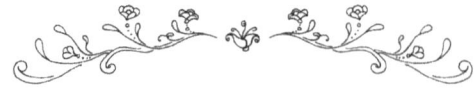

Minestrone
9, 1 cup servings - 151 calories each

2 Tbsp	extra-virgin olive oil
1/4	medium red onion, chopped
2	stalks celery, chopped
1/2 tsp	minced garlic
2 cups	water
4 cups	chicken broth
1 28 ounce	can whole plum tomatoes with juice, crushed with your hands
2	medium zucchini, coarsely chopped
6	baby carrots, sliced into 1/4 inch pieces
1 15 ounce	can cannellini beans, drained and rinsed
1/2 tsp	dried basil
1/2 tsp	salt
1/4 tsp	ground black pepper
5 ounces	fresh spinach

In a medium size soup pot over high heat combine olive oil, onion, celery and garlic. Saute until tender, approximately 2 to 3 minutes. Add water, broth, tomatoes, zucchini, carrots, beans, basil, salt and pepper. Cover and bring to a boil. Reduce heat to gently simmer for 1 hour. Add spinach and simmer 10 minutes more until spinach wilts.

ENJOY!

Roasted Minestrone
<u>12, 1 cup servings - 108 calories each</u>

1 large	baking potato, peeled and cubed
1 medium	eggplant, peeled and cubed
1	red pepper, cored, cut into 1/4 inch strips
1 medium	zucchini, stemmed, sliced into 1/2 inch discs
1/4 cup	extra-virgin olive oil, divided
4	plum tomatoes, cored, seeded, chopped
1 tsp	dried basil
1/4	medium red onion, chopped
2	cloves garlic, minced
2	stalks celery, chopped
4 cups	chicken broth
2 cups	water
1 28 ounce	can plum tomatoes, with juice, crushed with your hands
1/2 tsp	dried oregano
1/4 tsp	salt
1/2 tsp	ground black pepper

Preheat oven to 450 degrees.

Place potato, eggplant, red pepper and zucchini in a roasting pan with a cover. Drizzle with half of the olive oil. Cover and roast 20 minutes. Season the tomatoes with the dried basil and set aside. After the vegetables have roasted 20 minutes, add the tomatoes and continue to roast 10 minutes.

Meanwhile, in a large soup pot over medium heat, place remaining olive oil, onion, garlic and celery. Saute 5 minutes until vegetables are tender but not browned. Add broth, water, plum tomatoes with juice, oregano, salt and pepper. Increase the heat and bring to a boil. Adjust the heat to simmer gently.

Roasted Minestrone
continued

Remove the skins from the roasted tomatoes and add all of the roasted vegetables to the soup. Cover and gently simmer soup at least 30 minutes.

ENJOY!

Mom's Chicken Soup with My Twist
8, 1 cup servings broth - 10 calories each
2 cups broth with 2 meatballs - 90 calories

3 - 4 pound	whole chicken with giblets
1 tsp	salt
2 Tbsp	whole peppercorns
2 Tbsp	whole mustard seeds
1	bay leaf
1	stalk celery
1	carrot or 6 baby carrots
1/2 medium	red onion
1 Tbsp	dried parsley
1 recipe	Vegetable Meatballs (see following recipe)

Place chicken and giblets in a 6 quart soup pot. Cover chicken with 14 cups cold water. Add salt. Cover pot and bring to a boil. Reduce heat to simmer broth for 1 hour. Vent cover slightly while broth simmers.

Wrap the peppercorns, mustard seeds and bay leaf in cheesecloth and tie it closed. Alternatively, place the seasonings in a tea infuser. Add the seasonings, 2 cups water, the celery, carrot, onion and parsley to the soup. Simmer, undisturbed, 3 hours until chicken is tender. As the soup cooks, skim the scum off the surface. When the chicken is tender, remove it to a separate bowl with the vegetables. Discard the seasonings. Add 2 more cups of hot water and simmer 10 minutes.

Use the chicken for sandwiches, salads or in the soup as an alternative to the Vegetable Meatballs.

ENJOY!

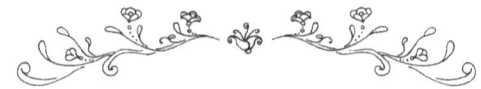

Vegetable Meatballs
17 meatballs - 35 calories each

3 cups	frozen, chopped spinach, thawed
1 cup	raw sweet potato, shredded
1 cup	raw zucchini, shredded
1 cup	raw red onion, shredded
8 Tbsp	uncooked Farina cereal
1/8 cup	egg substitute
1/4 tsp	salt
1/4 tsp	ground black pepper

Preheat oven to 375 degrees. Spray a baking pan with non-stick cooking spray. Set aside.

Thoroughly squeeze the water out of the spinach. Combine all the ingredients in a large bowl. Using your hands, mix well so that all the ingredients are distributed well. Form 17 meatballs and set them in the baking pan.

Bake for 15 minutes. Turn the meatballs over and bake for 15 minutes more.

In addition to adding the meatballs to Mom's Chicken Soup, they are also delicious served with a tomato sauce.

ENJOY!

Beans 'n Greens Soup
8 servings - 103 calories each

2 Tbsp	extra-virgin olive oil
1/4 cup	red onion, chopped
1	stalk celery, chopped
1	garlic clove, minced
1 medium	head escarole, cored, coarsely chopped
3 cups	spinach, coarsely chopped
6 cups	chicken broth
5 cups	water
1 15 ounce	can cannellini beans, drained, rinsed
1/4 tsp	salt
1/8 tsp	ground black pepper
1/4 tsp	crushed rosemary
1/8 tsp	crushed red pepper flakes
12	cherry or grape tomatoes, halved

In a large soup pot, combine olive oil, onion, celery and garlic. Saute over medium heat 3 to 5 minutes until tender but not browned. Add escarole and spinach. Pour the broth and water over the greens. Cover and continue cooking over medium heat until the greens wilt, approximately 10 minutes.

Add the beans, salt, pepper, rosemary and red pepper flakes. Simmer on low 15 minutes. Add tomatoes and simmer an additional 5 minutes or until beans are heated through and tomatoes are softened.

ENJOY!

Pasta e Fagioli
6 servings - 252 calories each

1 Tbsp	extra-virgin olive oil
1 tsp	minced garlic
1/4 medium	red onion, chopped
1/4 medium	head of cabbage, chopped
2 cups	chicken broth
1 14 ounce	can crushed tomatoes with juice
1 15 ounce	can cannellini beans, drained and rinsed
1/4 tsp	ground black pepper
3/4 cup	ditalini or other small shaped pasta

Place olive oil, garlic and onion in a large soup pot over medium heat. Stir and saute for 3 to 4 minutes until translucent. Add the cabbage and 1 cup of water. Stir and cover. Simmer for 3 minutes until the cabbage is slightly wilted. Add broth, tomatoes, including juice, 1 tomato can of water, beans and pepper. Bring to a boil, stirring occasionally. Reduce heat and simmer, covered, 10 to 15 minutes.

Meanwhile, cook pasta according to package directions until al dente. Serve each bowl of soup with approximately 1/8 cup of pasta.

A 10 ounce package of fresh spinach can be substituted for the cabbage and garbanzo beans can be substituted for the cannellini beans.

ENJOY!

Vegetable Stew
6, 1 cup servings - 177 calories each

1/4 cup	dried porcini mushrooms
4	plum tomatoes
4 cups	chicken broth
1 medium	zucchini, stem and end removed
1 medium	yellow squash, stem and end removed
1 medium	eggplant, peeled
1/2 cup	dried lentil beans, rinsed and sorted
1 tsp	dried basil
1 tsp	dried oregano
1 tsp	salt
1/4 tsp	ground black pepper
1	bay leaf
1/2 head	escarole, rinsed well and chopped
2 cups	fresh spinach, rinsed well and chopped
1 18 ounce	tube prepared polenta

Place mushrooms in a small bowl and cover with hot water. Set aside 30 minutes. Core the tomatoes and cut an "x" in the bottom of each one.

In a large soup pot, bring the chicken broth to a boil. Gently lower the tomatoes into broth and simmer for 2 minutes. Remove the tomatoes and set aside to cool. When cool enough to handle, remove the skins and chop them.

Meanwhile, cut the zucchini lengthwise into quarters. Slice the quarters into 1/2 inch pieces. Do the same with the yellow squash and the eggplant.

Vegetable Stew
continued

Drain the mushrooms, rinse well and coarsely chop them. Place the mushrooms, tomatoes, zucchini, yellow squash, eggplant and lentils in the broth. Season with the basil, oregano, salt, pepper and bay leaf. Bring to a boil, cover and cook 10 minutes.

Add the escarole and spinach. Stir, cover and simmer 15 minutes. Cut the polenta into 6 slices. Stir the stew and smooth the top. Set the polenta slices on top of the stew. Cover and simmer 15 to 20 minutes until the polenta is heated through.

ENJOY!

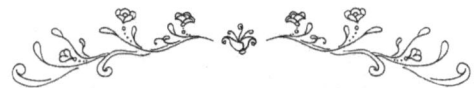

Thanksgiving Chili
<u>12 servings - 192 calories each</u>

1 pound	piece fresh pumpkin, seeds and pulp removed, but skin intact
2 Tbsp	extra-virgin olive oil
1 clove	garlic, minced
1 small	red onion, chopped
1 medium	green pepper, chopped
1 28 ounce	can plum tomatoes with juice, chopped
4 cups	chicken broth
1 15 ounce	can cannellini beans, drained and rinsed
2-1/2 cups	cooked turkey, cubed
2 tsp	dried parsley
1-1/2 tsp	dried oregano
1 tsp	crushed red pepper flakes
1/2 tsp	salt

Place pumpkin in a microwave-safe bowl. Cover with 1 inch water. Microwave on high 5 to 8 minutes or until pumpkin is tender but firm.

In a large soup pot combine olive oil, garlic, onion and green pepper. Saute over medium heat 3 to 4 minutes until tender. Add tomatoes with juice, broth, beans and 2 cups water. Increase heat to high and bring to a boil. Adjust heat to simmer gently.

When pumpkin is cool enough to handle, remove skin and cut flesh into 1 inch cubes. Add pumpkin, turkey, parsley, oregano, red pepper flakes and salt to chili and simmer gently, uncovered, 30 to 45 minutes.

Thanksgiving Chili
continued

Acorn squash or sweet potato can be substituted for the pumpkin. Precook acorn squash the same as pumpkin. If using sweet potato, peel, cube and add to pot with broth.

ENJOY!

Italian Chili
14 servings, 1 cup chili and 1/4 cup pasta
341 calories each

1 pound	bulk Italian sausage
2 slices	pancetta, chopped
1/2 cup	red onion, chopped
1/2 cup	green pepper, chopped
1	clove garlic, minced
1/2 cup	dry red wine
1 28 ounce	can plum tomatoes
1 28 ounce	can tomato puree
4 cups	water
1/4 tsp	crushed red pepper flakes
1 tsp	dried basil
1 tsp	dried oregano
1 pound	box ditalini pasta
1 15 ounce	can cannellini beans, rinsed and drained
1 15 ounce	can garbanzo beans, rinsed and drained
1/2 cup	part-skim shredded mozzarella cheese

In a large soup pot over medium-high heat, brown the sausage breaking it into medium size pieces as it browns. Remove the sausage to a strainer and set aside to drain the fat. To the same pot, add the pancetta, onion, green pepper and garlic. Saute 5 minutes until pancetta is brown and vegetables are tender. Add the wine and de-glaze the pot scraping the brown bits loose. Crush the plum tomatoes with your hands and add to the pot with the tomato puree, water, red pepper flakes, basil, oregano and drained sausage. Bring to a gentle simmer and cook 20 minutes.

Italian Chili
continued

Meanwhile, cook the pasta according to package directions until al dente. Drain pasta and rinse under cold water. Set aside to drain well.

Add the garbanzo and cannellini beans to the chili. Gently simmer until heated through, 10 to 15 minutes.

Use the mozzarella to sprinkle on each serving.

ENJOY!

Cabbage, Mushroom and Pork Soup
6 servings - 192 calories each

1	clove garlic, minced
1 Tbsp	extra-virgin olive oil
1 pound	pork tenderloin, trimmed of fat and gristle, cut into 1 inch pieces
1/2 tsp	ground sage
1/2 tsp	salt
1/2 tsp	ground black pepper
1/2 medium	head of cabbage, chopped
6 cups	chicken broth, divided
1 16 ounce	package while mushrooms, chopped
2 cups	hot water

Heat the oil and garlic in a large soup pot over medium heat. Saute 1 minute. Add the pork, sage, salt and pepper. Cook, stirring frequently, until pork is browned. Add the cabbage and 1/2 of the broth. Cook, stirring frequently, until the cabbage is wilted.

Add the remaining broth, mushrooms and water. Bring to a boil. Reduce heat to simmer gently, covered, about 30 minutes.

ENJOY!

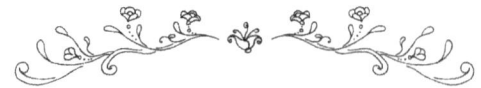

3 Days After the Pot Roast Soup
6, 1-1/2 cup servings - 128 calories each

6 cups	chicken broth
4 cups	water
4	plum tomatoes
2 stalks	celery, sliced
1/4	red onion, chopped
1/2 tsp	ground black pepper
1 tsp	dried basil
2 servings	leftover pot roast with vegetables (see recipe Slow Cooker Italian Beef Roast)
2 cups	fresh spinach, coarsely chopped

Combine chicken broth and water in a large soup pot and bring to a boil. Meanwhile, remove cores from tomatoes and make and "x" shaped cut in the bottom of each. When the broth comes to a boil, carefully lower tomatoes into broth. Remove the tomatoes after 1 minute. When cool enough to handle, peel the skin off the tomatoes. Chop the tomatoes and place back into the broth. Add the celery, onion, ground black pepper and basil. Gently stir and bring soup to a boil. Lower heat to simmer and cook for 1 hour.

Coarsely chop the pot roast and vegetables. Add the meat, vegetables and spinach to the soup. Stir and gently simmer 45 minutes.

ENJOY!

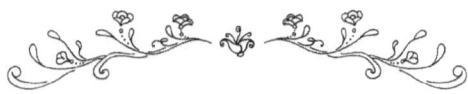

Main Dishes

Marinated Salmon Fillet
Roasted Red Snapper
Citrus Roasted Fish
Tuna and Vegetable Lasagna
Slow Cooker Roast Chicken
Slow Cooker Pot Roast
Slow Cooker Italian Beef Roast
Meatloaf
Sausage Meatballs
Braised Sausage Stew
Corn Dog Casserole
Tuscan Tamales
New Year's Day Pasta e Lenticchie
Tortellini with Zucchini and Tomato
Individual Vegetarian "Casseroles"
Stuffed Eggplant
Stuffed Acorn Squash
Stuffed Pumpkin

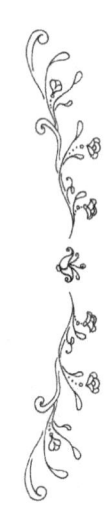

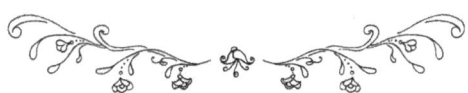

Marinated Salmon Fillet
6, 8 ounce servings - 408 calories each

3 pound	salmon fillet
10 Tbsp	lemon juice
1 cup	orange juice
2 cups	dry white wine
4 sprigs	fresh Italian parsley
2 tsp	dried chives
2 tsp	dried dill
1/3 cup	honey
1/4 tsp	salt
1/2 cup	extra-virgin olive oil

Arrange salmon fillet in a large cooking bag so it is flat. Set the bag on a baking sheet. Place the lemon and orange juices, white wine, parsley, chives, dill, honey and salt in the bowl of a food processor. Process while adding the olive oil for 1 minute or until the mixture is emulsified. Depending on the size of your processor, you may need to do this in batches.

Pour the marinade over the salmon. Twist tie the opening closed. Set in the refrigerator to marinate for 48 hours. While marinating turn the bag over 3 or 4 times and massage the fillet.

If you prefer your salmon less pink in the center as I do, before serving, transfer salmon to a roasting pan, drizzle with 1/2 cup of the marinade and roast at 350 degrees for 15 minutes.

ENJOY!

Roasted Red Snapper
4 servings - 281 calories each

3 Tbsp	extra-virgin olive oil, divided
1 medium	fennel bulb, thinly sliced
1 1-1/2 lb.	whole red snapper, gutted and scaled
1/2 tsp	minced garlic
1/4 tsp	salt
1/4 tsp	ground black pepper
2 tsp	lemon juice
1 tsp	dried rosemary
1 tsp	dried thyme
1 small	orange, thinly sliced

Preheat oven to 400 degrees.

Spread 1 Tbsp olive oil on the inside of a piece of aluminum foil large enough to loosely envelope the fish. Lay the sliced fennel across the middle of the foil. Wash the inside and outside of the fish with cold water and pat dry with a paper towel. Lay the fish on top of the fennel. Spread the garlic in the cavity of the fish. Season the inside and outside with salt and pepper. Drizzle inside and outside with the remaining olive oil and lemon juice and gently massage them into the fish.

Wrap the rosemary and thyme in cheesecloth and set inside the cavity. Lay half of the orange slices on the fish. Loosely seal the edges of the aluminum foil.

Roast 35 to 40 minutes or until the fish is cooked through at the bone and the fish flakes easily with a fork.

Roasted Red Snapper
continued

With a sharp knife, separate the two fillets from the backbone. With a spatula, remove the top fillet to the serving platter. Lift off the head and backbone and discard. Add the bottom fillets to the serving platter and garnish with the remaining orange slices.

ENJOY!

Citrus Roasted Fish
4 servings - 246 calories each

1	orange, thinly sliced
4 - 5 ounce	fish fillets such as cod, salmon or tuna
1/2 tsp	salt
1/2 tsp	ground black pepper
1/2 tsp	dried oregano
1	clove garlic, minced

Preheat oven to 425 degrees. Spray a roasting pan with butter flavored non-stick cooking spray.

Lay the orange slices in the bottom of the pan. Lay the fish fillets on top of the orange slices. Season the fish with the salt, pepper, oregano and garlic. Cover the roasting pan with aluminum foil.

Roast 30 to 35 minutes or until fish is cooked through and flakes easily with a fork.

ENJOY!

Tuna and Vegetable Lasagna
6 servings - 310 calories each

1 medium	eggplant
	salt
6	lasagna noodles
2 medium	zucchini
1/8 cup	extra-virgin olive oil
1 6 ounce	can Italian tuna packed in olive oil
1 6 ounce	can solid albacore tuna in water, drained
1/4 tsp	ground black pepper
1 12 ounce	jar roasted red peppers
2 large	tomatoes
1 Tbsp	fresh basil, chopped
1/2 cup	shredded part-skim mozzarella
2 Tbsp	grated Romano cheese
1 cup	chicken broth

Peel eggplant and slice crosswise into 1/8 " slices. Layer slices in a colander, lightly salting each layer. Set aside 30 minutes.

Cook the lasagna noodles according to package directions until very al dente. Rinse, drain and set aside.

Preheat oven to 400 degrees. Spray 2 baking pans with non-stick cooking spray. Slice the zucchini lengthwise into 1/4 " slices. Place zucchini in 1 prepared baking pan. Drizzle with half the olive oil and roast for 10 minutes. Wipe the eggplant slices dry with paper towels and place in the second prepared baking pan. Drizzle with the remaining olive oil. After the zucchini have roasted 10 minutes, turn the slices over. Add the eggplant to the oven and roast for 15 minutes.

Tuna and Vegetable Lasagna
continued

Turn the eggplant over halfway through the cooking time.

Meanwhile, place the Italian tuna with olive oil and the drained albacore tuna in a medium bowl. Season with pepper. Stir to combine and set aside.

Remove the equivalent of 1 medium red pepper from the jar and slice into 1/4" strips. Set aside. Refrigerate the rest for another use.

Slice the tomatoes into 1/4" slices and sprinkle with the basil. Set aside.

Reduce oven temperature to 350 degrees. Spray a 9 x 13 baking dish with non-stick cooking spray. Place 2 lasagna noodles in the baking dish. Top with all of the tuna mixture, spreading it evenly on the noodles. Place 2 more noodles on the tuna. Lay all of the eggplant slices evenly on the noodles. Place half of the tomato slices on the eggplant followed by half of the red pepper strips. Place the remaining 2 noodles on the red peppers followed by the zucchini, the remaining tomatoes and red pepper. Sprinkle the mozzarella and Romano evenly on top. Pour the broth in the pan. Cover with foil and bake for 25 minutes. Remove the foil the last 10 minutes of cooking time.

ENJOY!

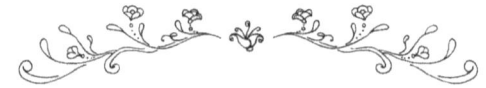

Slow Cooker Roast Chicken
6 servings - 212 calories each

3 - 3-1/2	pound whole chicken, skin and fat removed
1/2 tsp	salt
1/2 tsp	ground black pepper
1 tsp	crushed, dried rosemary
1/2	medium cabbage, cored, coarsely chopped
3 cups	water
1	1 pound package potato gnocchi
12	white or baby portobello mushrooms, halved

Spray inside of a 5 to 6 quart slow cooker with non-stick cooking spray.

Wash chicken inside and outside. Season inside and outside of chicken with salt, pepper and rosemary. Set in refrigerator while you prepare cabbage.

Lay cabbage in slow cooker and set chicken on top of cabbage. Add water to cooker. Cover cooker and cook on low 4 to 4-1/2 hours.

Add gnocchi and mushrooms to cooker for the last hour of cooking time, arranging the gnocchi so they are in the cooking liquid and the mushrooms on top of the gnocchi.

ENJOY!

Slow Cooker Pot Roast
6 servings - 280 calories each

1 14 ounce	sweet potato, peeled, quartered, cut into 1/2 inch slices
1/2	fennel bulb, coarsely chopped
1/4	red onion, coarsely chopped
12	baby carrots
4	plum tomatoes, halved, coarsely chopped
2 - 2-1/2	pound boneless beef chuck pot roast, trimmed of fat and gristle
1/2 tsp	dried basil
1/2 tsp	salt
1/2 tsp	ground black pepper
1 Tbsp	balsamic vinegar
1 cup	water

Spray inside of a 5 to 6 quart slow cooker with non-stick cooking spray. Lay sweet potato, fennel, onion, carrots and tomatoes in slow cooker. Rinse roast and dry with a paper towel. Season with basil, salt and pepper, massaging the seasonings into the meat. Lay the roast on top of the vegetables. Combine balsamic and water and pour over the roast.

Cover and cook on low 8 hours or on high 4 hours until beef is tender.

ENJOY!

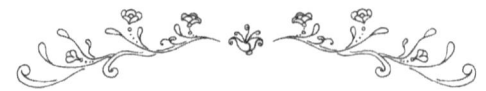

Slow Cooker Italian Beef Roast
6 servings - 307 calories each

2 pounds	top round steak
3/4 tsp	salt
1/2 tsp	ground black pepper
1/4 tsp	dried basil
1/4 tsp	dried oregano
1/4 tsp	crushed, dried rosemary
1	clove garlic, minced
6	red potatoes
12	baby carrots
1 cup	water
1 medium	zucchini

Rinse meat and dry with a paper towel. Season each side of steak with half of the salt, pepper, basil, oregano and rosemary. Press garlic into top side of meat. Set aside.

Cut each potato in half. Lay potatoes and carrots in the slow cooker. Lay the meat on top of the vegetables. Pour the water over meat and vegetables. Cover the cooker and cook on low 8 hours.

Cut the zucchini into 6 pieces and add to the cooker during the last hour of cooking time. Remove the meat and let it set 10 minutes before slicing.

ENJOY!

Meatloaf
8 servings - 173 calories each

3 slices	rye bread, torn into small pieces
1/4 cup	skim milk
1 pound	ground turkey
1/2 pound	bulk Italian sausage
1/4 cup	egg substitute
1/2 tsp	salt
1/4 tsp	ground black pepper
1 tsp	dried parsley
1/2 tsp	dried oregano
1 medium	tomato, thinly sliced

Preheat oven to 350 degrees. Spray an 11 x 7 loaf pan with non-stick cooking spray. Set aside.

Place bread in a large mixing bowl. Pour the skim milk over. Add the turkey, Italian sausage, egg substitute, salt, pepper, parsley and oregano. Mix gently just until combined. Don't overwork the mixture. Form into a loaf and set the loaf into the prepared pan.

Lay the tomato slices on top of the meatloaf. Cover the pan with aluminum foil and bake for 35 minutes. Uncover the pan and bake for an additional 15 to 20 minutes until browned. Let stand 10 minutes before slicing.

ENJOY!

Sausage Meatballs
2 meatballs, 1 cup gravy - 301 calories

2 cups	beef broth, divided
1/2 tsp	minced garlic
1/2 tsp	ground black pepper, divided
2 cups	tomatoes, seeded and chopped
2 Tbsp	tomato paste
5	fresh basil leaves, torn
1 slice	day old country style Italian bread, torn into small pieces
1/4 cup	skim milk
1 pound	bulk Italian sausage
1 cup	romaine lettuce, torn into small pieces
1/4 cup	egg substitute
1/4 cup	grated Romano cheese

Combine 1/4 cup of beef broth and garlic in a medium soup pot and saute over medium-high heat until garlic is golden. Add the remaining beef broth and 1/4 tsp of pepper. Bring to a boil. Add the tomatoes and tomato paste and stir to dissolve the paste. Add the basil leaves and simmer gently while you prepare the meatballs.

Place the bread in a medium size bowl and pour the milk over. Toss the bread around gently so the milk moistens all of the bread. Place the sausage in a separate large bowl. Squeeze the bread out and add it to the sausage along with the lettuce, egg substitute, cheese and remaining 1/4 tsp of pepper. Stir the mixture together to evenly combine all the ingredients.

Sausage Meatballs
__continued__

Form 14 meatballs and add them to the gravy along with 2 cups hot water. Bring to a boil. Reduce heat to gently simmer 30 minutes or until meatballs are cooked through.

ENJOY!

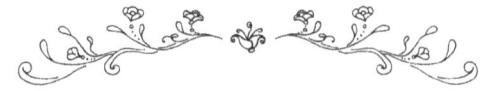

Braised Sausage Stew
6 servings - 375 calories each

2 cups	chicken broth
1/2 cup	Dijon mustard
2 Tbsp	honey
1/2 medium	head cabbage, coarsely chopped
1-1/4 pound	approx. 4 red potatoes, coarsely chopped
1 tsp	salt
1 tsp	ground black pepper
2 medium	apples, cored and coarsely chopped
1 14 ounce	package light smoked sausage

In a large soup pot over medium-high head, whisk together the chicken broth, Dijon and honey. Add the cabbage, potatoes, salt and pepper and stir. Cover and simmer 30 minutes. Add the apples and stir. Lay the sausage on top. Cover and continue to gently simmer 20 minutes until apples are crisp tender and sausage is heated through. To serve, cut the sausage into 6 pieces.

ENJOY!

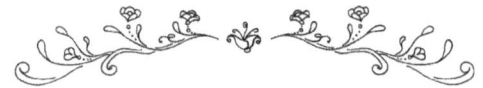

Corn Dog Casserole
8 servings - 319 calories each

4 cups	cold water
1 cup	instant polenta
1 tsp	salt
1 Tbsp	extra-virgin olive oil
1/2 cup	cheddar cheese, diced, divided
1/4 tsp	crushed red pepper flakes
1 package	beef hot dogs, cut into 1/4" slices
1/4 cup	prepared mustard

Spray an 8 x 8 casserole with non-stick butter flavored cooking spray. Set aside.

Combine the water, polenta, salt and olive oil in a large, deep sauce pot over medium-high head. Bring to a boil, stirring constantly with a wooden spoon. When the polenta starts to bubble, adjust the heat to simmer gently 3 minutes more, stirring constantly.

Remove from heat and fold in half of the cheddar cheese. Pour half of the polenta into the prepared casserole. Smooth the surface of the polenta. Evenly sprinkle the red pepper flakes over the polenta. Lay the hot dog slices on top of the polenta. Fold the prepared mustard into the remaining polenta distributing it well. Pour the polenta over the hot dogs and smooth the surface. Cover the casserole with plastic wrap and refrigerate 1 hour to firm the polenta.

Corn Dog Casserole
continued

Preheat oven to 375 degrees. Remove the plastic wrap and lightly brush to top with a little olive oil. Distribute the remaining cheddar evenly on top. Bake for 30 to 35 minutes until heated through.

ENJOY!

Tuscan Tamales
8 tamales - 166 calories each
1-3/4 cups sauce - 1/4 cup, 19 calories

1 28 ounce	can crushed tomatoes
1/4 tsp	granulated garlic
1/2 tsp	dried oregano
3/4 tsp	dried basil
1/8 tsp	crushed red pepper flakes
1/4 tsp	ground black pepper, divided
3-1/2 cups	cold water
1 cup	instant polenta or cornmeal
1 tsp	salt
1/2 cup	grated Parmigiano Reggiano
8 ounces	cooked chicken, shredded with a fork
4 cups	fresh spinach, chopped
1/2 tsp	crushed rosemary

Place the crushed tomatoes in a large bowl. Season with the garlic, oregano, basil, red pepper flakes and 1/8 tsp of black pepper. Stir well, cover and set aside.

Cut 8 squares of parchment paper approx. 8" x 8". Set aside.

Combine the water, polenta and salt in a large soup pot over medium-high heat. Bring to a boil, stirring constantly, with a wooden spoon. When the polenta starts to bubble, adjust the heat to simmer gently 3 minutes, stirring constantly. Remove from heat and stir in the Parmigiano.

Tuscan Tamales
<u>continued</u>

Spread a layer of polenta on each parchment paper approx. 1/8" thick and 4" x 4" square. Set aside.

Combine shredded chicken, chopped spinach, rosemary and the remaining 1/8 tsp of black pepper in a medium bowl. Mix well.

Lay the chicken mixture in a log shape down the center of each prepared polenta square, dividing it equally.

Working with one tamale at a time and starting at one long end, roll the cornmeal up around the filling. Slide the tamale to the bottom edge of the parchment and roll the parchment up around the tamale. Twist each end closed. Repeat for the remaining tamales.

To heat the tamales, steam them by placing the tamales in a steamer basket over approx. 2" of water in a large soup pot. Steam for 20 to 25 minutes or until heated through. Alternatively, lay the tamales in a microwave-save bowl with approx. 1" of water and microwave on high 5 minutes or until heated through.

Heat the sauce either stovetop or in the microwave.

ENJOY!

New Year's Day Pasta e Lenticchie
8, 1 cup servings - 281 calories each

1/2 cup	sun dried tomatoes (not in oil)
1 48 ounce	can chicken broth
1 cup	dried lentils, sorted
1/4 tsp	ground black pepper
1/8 tsp	crushed red pepper flakes
1/4 tsp	granulated garlic
1 pound	ditalini or other small shaped pasta
8 Tbsp	grated Parmigiano Reggiano cheese

Snip tomatoes into strips and soak in hot water 15 minutes. Drain and set aside.

In a medium soup pot, combine tomatoes, chicken broth and lentils. Cover and simmer 30 minutes. Add two cups hot water, pepper, red pepper and garlic and simmer on low an additional 30 minutes.

Meanwhile, cook pasta according to package directions until al dente. Drain and rinse pasta.

To serve, place pasta in serving bowl, top with lentils and finish each with 1 Tbsp of cheese.

ENJOY!

Tortellini with Zucchini and Tomato
2 servings - 410 calories each

1-1/3 cup	cheese tortellini
1	garlic clove, minced
2 Tbsp	extra-virgin olive oil
1 medium	zucchini, chopped
3	plum tomatoes, chopped
2 Tbsp	grated Parmigiano Reggiano

Cook pasta according to package directions.

Meanwhile, combine olive oil and garlic in a medium saute pan. Saute garlic 1 minute. Add zucchini. Saute 4 to 5 minutes until lightly browned and crisp tender. Add tomato and saute 3 to 4 minutes.

When pasta is cooked, drain but reserve approximately 1 cup of the water. Add pasta to vegetables and gently stir together. Add 1 Tbsp each of the cheese and reserved pasta water. Gently stir. Continue to add the pasta water 1 Tbsp at a time until a creamy texture is achieved. Serve topped with the remaining 1 Tbsp of cheese.

ENJOY!

Individual Vegetarian "Casseroles"
2 servings - 153 calories each

1 medium	eggplant, peeled and diced
1	zucchini, diced
6	mushrooms, sliced
1 medium	red pepper, seeded and diced
1/2 tsp	salt
1/2 tsp	ground black pepper
1 tsp	dried basil
1/2 cup	fat-free ricotta cheese
1/8 tsp	granulated garlic
1/8 tsp	salt
1/8 tsp	ground black pepper
1/4 tsp	dried oregano

Preheat oven to 425 degrees.

Make 4 pieces of aluminum foil 12" x 12" and spray 1 side of each with non-stick cooking spray. On each of 2 pieces of foil, layer half of the eggplant, zucchini, mushrooms and red pepper. Season each with half of the 1/2 tsp salt, 1/2 tsp pepper and 1 tsp basil.

In a small bowl, combine the ricotta, garlic, 1/8 tsp salt, 1/8 tsp pepper and 1/4 tsp oregano and mix well. Dollop half of the ricotta mixture on each "casserole."

Lay 1 of the remaining pieces of foil on top of each "casserole" and tightly pinch all four sides together. Bake 50 to 55 minutes.

ENJOY!

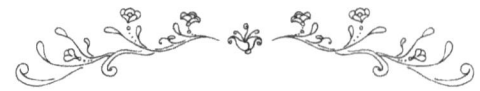

Stuffed Eggplant
2 servings - 159 calories each

1 medium	eggplant
1 cup	fat-free ricotta cheese
1	clove garlic, minced
1/4 tsp	salt
1/8 tsp	ground black pepper
1/2 tsp	dried oregano
1	plum tomato, cored, seeded, cut lengthwise into 8 thin slices
1/4 tsp	dried basil
1 tsp	grated Romano cheese

Remove stem of eggplant and cut eggplant in half.

Being careful not to pierce the skin, make 3 to 4 slits in the flesh to form pockets for the stuffing. In a microwave-safe bowl large enough to hold both halves, add the eggplant and approximately 1" of water. Cover the bowl with microwave-safe plastic wrap. Vent the cover. Microwave on high approximately 8 minutes or until eggplant is tender.

Lay eggplant halves, cut side down on paper towels to dry. Set aside to cool.

Meanwhile, combine ricotta, garlic, salt, pepper and oregano. Mix well.

Preheat oven to 350 degrees.

Stuffed Eggplant
continued

When eggplant is cool, divide the cheese mixture evenly between the two halves, spooning it into the slits. Top each with half of the tomato slices. Sprinkle each with half of the basil and cheese.

Bake for approximately 30 minutes or until cheese is bubbly and tomatoes are lightly browned.

ENJOY!

Stuffed Acorn Squash
2 servings - 323 calories each

1 medium	acorn squash, halved, seeded, cleaned
1 cup	fresh butternut squash, peeled, cubed
1 medium	apple, cored and cubed
2	dried apricots, diced
4 ounces	cooked turkey breast, cubed
1/4 tsp	salt
1/4 tsp	ground black pepper
1/2 tsp	crushed dried rosemary, divided
3/4 Tbsp	honey

Place acorn squash cut sides down in a microwave-safe baking dish. Arrange squash cubes around the acorn halves. Microwave, uncovered, on high approximately 15 minutes until tender.

Meanwhile, in a large bowl, combine the apple cubes, apricots, turkey, salt pepper and 1/4 tsp of the rosemary. Mix well and set aside.

Preheat oven to 325 degrees. Spray an oven-safe baking dish with non-stick cooking spray. When the squash is tender, transfer the halves , cut sides up, to the prepared baking dish. Drizzle half of the honey over each and sprinkle each with half of the remaining rosemary. Add the squash cubes to the apple mixture and mix well.

Fill each acorn cavity with the apple mixture. Arrange any remaining apple mixture in the baking dish around the halves. Bake 20 minutes. Increase temperature to 375 degrees and bake 20 to 25 minutes more.

ENJOY!

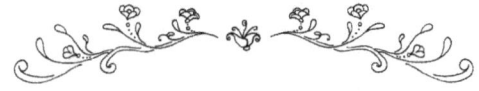

Stuffed Pumpkin
2 servings - 380 calories each

1 cup	fresh cranberries, rinsed and drained
1 tsp	honey
1 medium	pie pumpkin
1/2 tsp	salt
1/4 tsp	ground black pepper
1/2 tsp	ground cinnamon
8 ounces	cooked turkey breast, cubed
1/4 tsp	salt
1/8 tsp	ground black pepper
1/2 tsp	crushed dried rosemary

Coarsely chop the cranberries in a food processor. Transfer the cranberries to a large mixing bowl. Add the honey and mix well. Set aside. Preheat oven to 375 degrees.

Core pumpkin. Cut pumpkin in half and remove the seeds. Lay the halves in a microwave-safe bowl cut sides up and add approximately 2" of water. Microwave on high 10 minutes. Drain the water and set pumpkin aside.

Spray a baking pan with non-stick cooking spray. Set the pumpkin halves in the pan. Season each with 1/4 tsp salt, 1/8 tsp pepper and 1/4 tsp cinnamon.

To the cranberry mixture add the turkey, the 1/4 tsp salt, 1/8 tsp pepper and 1/2 tsp rosemary. Mix well. Evenly divide the cranberry mixture between the two pumpkin halves. Bake for 20 to 25 minutes.

ENJOY!

Side Dishes

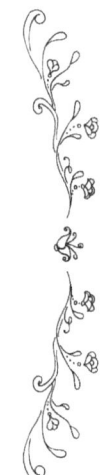

Spinach and Escarole Saute
Steamed Greens and 'Shrooms
Cheesy Spinach
Roasted Vegetable Packets
Fresh Balsamic Green Beans
Special Green Beans
Grilled Eggplant
Sweet Sour Beet Salad
Zucchini Cranberry Salad
Cole Slaw 1
Cole Slaw 2
Quick Coleslaw
Cheesy Potato Salad
Italian Potato Salad
Cooking Fresh Squash
Cannellini Bean Salad
Honey and Cinnamon Apple Saute

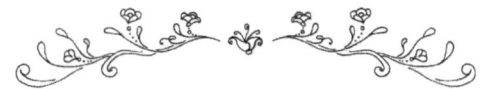

Spinach and Escarole Saute
4 servings - 101 calories each

2 Tbsp	extra-virgin olive oil
1	garlic clove
2 medium	tomatoes, chopped
2 bunches	escarole, core removed
10 ounces	fresh spinach
1/4 tsp	salt
1/4 tsp	ground black pepper

Gently crush the garlic clove with the side of a knife to release the flavor. Place the garlic clove and olive oil in a large soup pot. Gently saute for 1 minute. Remove the garlic clove.

Add tomatoes and continue to saute for 3 minutes. Rinse escarole and spinach and add to pot with the water still clinging to the leaves. Add salt and pepper and stir. Cover pot and simmer 10 to 12 minutes, stirring occasionally, until the greens are wilted.

A medium size bunch of kale can be substituted for the spinach.

ENJOY!

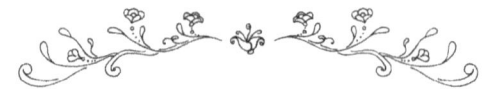

Steamed Greens and 'Shrooms
2 servings - 140 calories each

10 ounces	fresh spinach
1 bunch	escarole, core removed
1/4 tsp	salt
1/8 tsp	ground black pepper
8	white mushrooms, halved
2 tsp	extra-virgin olive oil

Thoroughly rinse the spinach and escarole. Place greens in a large soup pot with the water still clinging to the leaves. Add 1/2 cup water. Season with salt and pepper and toss the greens to distribute the seasoning. Set the mushrooms on top of the greens Cover the pot and steam over medium-high heat approximately 15 minutes or until the greens are wilted.

At serving time, drizzle 1 tsp olive oil over each serving.

ENJOY!

Cheesy Spinach
2 servings - 95 calories each

1/4 cup	fat-free ricotta cheese
1/16 tsp	granulated garlic
1/8 tsp	salt
1/8 tsp	ground black pepper
1/8 tsp	dried oregano
1 tsp	extra-virgin olive oil
1	garlic clove, minced
1/4 medium	red onion, chopped
2	plum tomatoes, cored, seeded, chopped
1 10 ounce	bag fresh spinach

In a small bowl, combine ricotta, granulated garlic, salt, pepper and oregano. Mix well and set aside.

Spray a large soup pot with non-stick, butter flavored cooking spray. Add olive oil, garlic clove and onion. Over medium heat, gently saute 1 minute until tender. Add tomatoes, spinach and 1 Tbsp of water. Cover pot and cook approximately 2 minutes to wilt spinach. Add ricotta mixture and stir to combine. Gently simmer approximately 2 minutes to heat cheese through.

ENJOY!

Roasted Vegetable Packets
<u>2 servings - 98 calories each</u>

2 cups	fresh spinach
1 medium	zucchini
6 mini	sweet peppers or 2 medium red peppers
2 medium	tomatoes
1 tsp	salt
1/2 tsp	ground black pepper
1 tsp	dried basil
1 tsp	dried oregano

Preheat oven to 425 degrees. Cut 2 pieces of aluminum foil approximately 16" x 16". Spray with non-stick cooking spray.

Lay 1 cup of spinach in the center of each piece of foil. Cut the zucchini into quarters lengthwise, then slice crosswise into 1/2" pieces. Set half of the zucchini on top of each pile of spinach. Core and seed the peppers and slice them into 1/2" pieces. Place 1/2 of the peppers in each packet. Core and seed the tomatoes. Chop them and add 1/2 the tomatoes to each packet. Season each with half of the salt, pepper, basil and oregano.

Tightly seal each packet. roast for 30 to 40 minutes until vegetables are crisp tender.

ENJOY!

Fresh Balsamic Green Beans
2 servings - 82 calories each

3/4 pound	fresh green beans (approx. 60 beans)
1-1/2 Tbsp	balsamic vinegar
1 tsp	honey
1/4 tsp	salt
1/8 tsp	ground black pepper
1/8 tsp	dried oregano
1/8 tsp	dried basil
1/16 tsp	crushed rosemary
2 tsp	grated Romano cheese

Trim the ends of green beans and, if desired, cut them in half. Place the beans in a microwave-safe bowl and cover them with water. Microwave on high 8 to 10 minutes or until crisp tender.

Meanwhile, in a small microwave-save bowl, whisk together the vinegar, honey, salt, pepper, oregano, basil and rosemary. Set aside.

When the green beans are at the desired crisp tenderness, drain them and return them to the cooking bowl. Sprinkle on the Romano cheese.

Microwave the vinegar mixture on high 1 minute. Pour the vinegar over the beans and toss to coat.

ENJOY!

Special Green Beans
4 servings - 136 calories each

3/4 pound	fresh green beans (approx. 60 beans)
1/8 tsp	salt
1 medium	apple, cored and chopped
2 Tbsp	walnut halves, coarsely chopped
1/8 cup	honey
1/8 cup	gorgonzola cheese

Preheat oven to 425 degrees. Spray a baking pan with non-stick cooking spray.

Trim the ends from the green beans and, if desired, cut the beans in half. Place the beans in the prepared baking pan. Spray the beans with butter flavored non-stick cooking spray. Sprinkle with salt. Toss the beans to distribute the salt and arrange them in a single layer. Roast for 15 minutes.

Add the chopped apples to the beans and toss to evenly combine the apples with the beans. Roast 15 minutes or until the beans and apples are tender.

Add the walnuts to the pan and drizzle the honey over the mixture. Stir gently to evenly coat.

At serving time, crumble the gorgonzola on each serving, dividing it equally.

ENJOY!

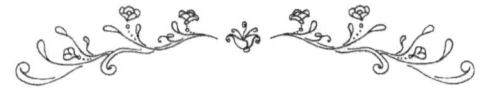

Grilled Eggplant
2 servings - 110 calories each

1 medium	eggplant
1/4 cup	fat-free ricotta cheese
1 Tbsp	balsamic vinegar
1/4 tsp	dried basil
1/4 tsp	dried oregano
1/8 tsp	granulated garlic
1/4 tsp	salt
1/4 tsp	ground black pepper
2 Tbsp	grated Parmigiano Reggiano

Remove the stem and peel from the eggplant. Cut the eggplant into 8 1" thick slices. Spray both sides of eggplant with non-stick cooking spray and arrange slices in a single layer on a baking sheet. Broil eggplant slices 7 to 10 minutes.

Meanwhile, in a small bowl, combine the ricotta, balsamic, basil, oregano, garlic, salt and pepper. Remove the eggplant from the broiler and turn the slices over. Lightly brush each slice with the ricotta mixture. Broil an additional 7 to 10 minutes until the cheese is browned and eggplant is tender.

While the eggplant is still hot, sprinkle on the grated Parmigiano.

ENJOY!

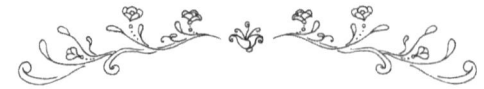

Sweet Sour Beet Salad
4 servings - 114 calories each

2 large	beets, 16 to 18 ounces total
1	apple, cored and chopped
1	orange, peeled and chopped
1/4 tsp	dried dill
1 tsp	honey
2 Tbsp	cider vinegar

Preheat oven to 450 degrees.

Place 1/2 cup water in a baking pan. Set the beets in pan and cover pan tightly with aluminum foil. Roast 1 hour or until beets are easily pierced with a fork. Drain water from pan and set beets aside to cool.

When the beets are cool enough to handle, trim off the roots and stems. Rub the skins off under running water. Chop the beets.

Combine the beets, apple, orange,dill, honey and cider vinegar. Mix well. Refrigerate at least 1 hour before serving.

ENJOY!

Zucchini Cranberry Salad
4 servings - 76 calories each

1 tsp	reduced-fat mayonnaise
1 Tbsp	fat-free sour cream
2 tsp	cider vinegar
3/4 tsp	honey
2 medium	zucchini, cut into matchstick size pieces
1/8 medium	red onion, cut into thin slivers
1/4 cup	dried cranberries
1/4 tsp	salt
1/8 tsp	ground black pepper

In a medium size bowl, whisk together the mayonnaise, sour cream, cider vinegar and honey. Add the zucchini, onion and cranberries and season with salt and pepper.
Mix well to combine.

Refrigerate 1 hour before serving.

ENJOY!

Cole Slaw 1
4, 1 cup servings - 57 calories each

1/2 cup	reduced-fat mayonnaise
1/2 cup	cider vinegar
1 tsp	honey
1-1/2 tsp	brown, grainy mustard
1 tsp	celery seed
1/8 tsp	salt
4 cups	cabbage, shredded (approx. 1/2 of a medium head)
1/2 cup	red bell pepper
1/4 cup	red onion, minced
1/4 tsp	salt
1/8 tsp	ground black pepper

In a large bowl, whisk together the mayonnaise, vinegar, honey, mustard, celery seed and 1/8 tsp salt. Add the cabbage, red pepper, red onion, 1/4 tsp salt and pepper.

Mix very well to evenly combine all the ingredients.

Refrigerate at least 1 hour before serving.

ENJOY!

Cole Slaw 2
4, 1 cup servings - 85 calories each

1/2 cup	fat-free sour cream
1 Tbsp	reduced-fat mayonnaise
1/4 cup	cider vinegar
1 tsp	honey
3 Tbsp	brown, grainy mustard
1/2 tsp	salt, divided
1/4 tsp	ground black pepper, divided
4 cups	cabbage, shredded (approx. 1/2 of a medium head)
1	apple, cored and diced
2	stalks celery, thinly sliced

In a large bowl, whisk together the sour cream, mayonnaise, vinegar, honey, mustard, 1/4 tsp salt and 1/8 tsp pepper.

Add the cabbage, apple, celery and the remaining 1/4 tsp salt and 1/8 tsp pepper.

Mix very well to evenly combine all the ingredients. Refrigerate at least 1 hour before serving.

A pear can be substituted for the apple.

ENJOY!

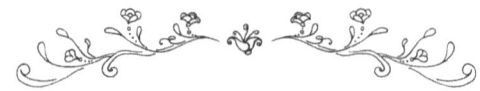

Quick Coleslaw
2 servings - 55 calories each

1/4 medium	head of cabbage, sliced very thin
2 Tbsp	red onion, minced
1/4 tsp	salt
1/8 tsp	ground black pepper
6 Tbsp	prepared fat-free Italian dressing

Place the cabbage and onion in a medium size bowl. Season with salt and pepper and stir. Pour the dressing over and stir very well.

Cover and refrigerate at least 1 hour before serving.

Stir well again before serving.

ENJOY!

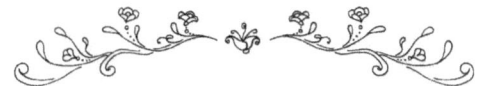

Cheesy Potato Salad
2 servings - 198 calories each

1 medium	baking potato
1/4 tsp	salt
1/8 tsp	ground black pepper
1 Tbsp	part-skim ricotta cheese
1 medium	stalk celery, thinly sliced
1 Tbsp	red onion, cut into thin slivers
5 medium	fresh basil leaves, cut into thin strips
1-1/2 Tbsp	extra-virgin olive oil
2 tsp	white balsamic vinegar

Preheat oven to 450 degrees. Wrap potato in aluminum foil and bake for 45 minutes or until a fork can easily pierce the center of the potato. Remove the foil and let the potato cool. When the potato is cool enough to handle but still slightly warm, dice it into 1" pieces and place in a medium size bowl. Season with salt and pepper.

Add ricotta and gently stir to combine. Add the celery, onion, basil, olive oil and balsamic. Stir again gently to distribute ingredients evenly and coat with olive oil.

ENJOY!

Italian Potato Salad
4 servings - 206 calories each

1 14 ounce	package potato gnocchi
1 Tbsp	white balsamic vinegar
1 Tbsp	Dijon mustard
1/8 tsp	granulated garlic
1/8 tsp	salt
1/8 tsp	ground black pepper
1/4 tsp	dried oregano
2 Tbsp	extra-virgin olive oil
1/8 cup	red onion, thinly sliced
1/4 medium	fennel bulb, thinly sliced
1 cup	grape tomatoes, halved
1 medium	stalk celery, thinly sliced
6	fresh basil leaves, thinly sliced

Place gnocchi in a large microwave-safe bowl. Cover gnocchi with 8 cups water. Microwave on high 10 minutes.
Stir halfway through cooking time. Drain and rinse well with cold water. Leave gnocchi in colander to drain well while cooling.

In the same cooking bowl, whisk together the vinegar, Dijon, garlic, salt, pepper and oregano. Continue whisking while adding the olive oil. Whisk until the dressing is emulsified. Add the gnocchi, red onion, fennel, tomatoes and celery to the dressing. Gently toss to coat the ingredients with the dressing. Sprinkle the basil on top.

Serve warm, room temperature or chilled.

ENJOY!

Cooking Fresh Squash
Pumpkin - 49 calories per cup
Butternut Squash - 82 calories per cup
Acorn Squash - 115 calories per cup

1	pie pumpkin
	or
1	butternut squash
	or
1	acorn squash

Core pumpkin or cut off stem end of butternut or acorn squash. Cut squash in half and scoop out the pulp and seeds. Soak or rinse the seeds and discard the pulp. Reserve the seeds for roasting. (See recipe "Roasted Squash Seeds").

Carve the squash into medium size wedges or pieces. Place 2" of water into a deep microwave-safe bowl. Place squash in bowl and cover with microwave-safe plastic wrap. Vent the plastic by cutting a couple of slits in the top.

If squash will be cubed for use in soups, stews or casseroles, microwave on high 6 to 8 minutes. If squash will be mashed or pureed, microwave on high 10 to 12 minutes. When the squash is cool enough to handle, remove the skin and prepare as desired.

ENJOY!

Cannellini Bean Salad
4 servings - 148 calories each

1 15 ounce	can cannellini beans, rinsed and drained
1 stalk	celery, thinly sliced
1 Tbsp	red onion, cut into thin slivers
1	plum tomato, seeded and chopped
1/2 tsp	salt
1/8 tsp	ground black pepper
1/2 tsp	dried oregano
1-1/2 Tbsp	extra-virgin olive oil
2 tsp	white balsamic vinegar

To a medium size bowl, add beans, celery, onion and tomato. Season with salt, pepper and oregano. Stir together. Add olive oil and balsamic and stir together.

Refrigerate 1 hour before serving.

Stir again before serving

ENJOY!

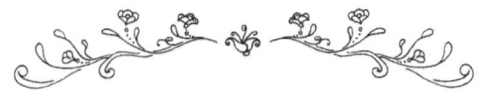

Honey and Cinnamon Apple Saute
4 servings - 117 calories each

1 tsp	butter
1/4 cup	apple juice
2 tsp	honey
1 tsp	lemon juice
1/2 tsp	ground cinnamon
1/8 tsp	salt
4 medium	apples, unpeeled, sliced into 1/2" thick wedges

Melt the butter in a medium size soup pot over medium heat. Add apple juice. Whisk in honey, lemon juice, cinnamon and salt. Simmer 1 minute. Add apples. Stir well to coat apples. Saute, covered, stirring occasionally, until apples are tender, approximately 15 minutes.

ENJOY!

Desserts and Beverages

Affogato
"Wine" and Cheese Rice Pudding
Peanutty Chocolate Covered Banana Parfait
Strawberries Italiano
Strawberries and Cream
Easy, Delicious Fresh Fruit Dessert
Mocha "Latte"

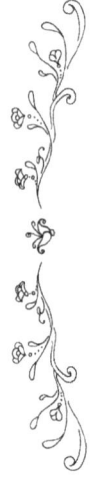
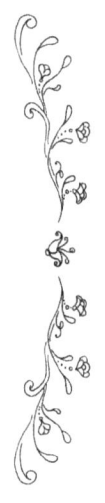

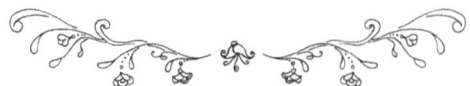

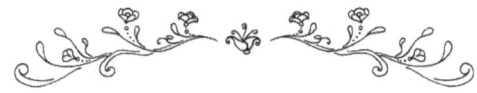

Affogato
1 serving - 99 calories each

1	fat-free frozen Greek yogurt bar
1/2 tsp	mini semi-sweet chocolate chips
1/8 cup	freshly brewed espresso or strong coffee

Cut the yogurt bar into 1" cubes and place in a 2 cup glass or parfait dish. Surround the yogurt cubes with the chocolate chips.

Slowly pour the hot coffee first over the chocolate chips to start melting them and then over the yogurt cubes.

As an option, serve with a biscotto to scoop up the yogurt. (calories not included).

ENJOY!

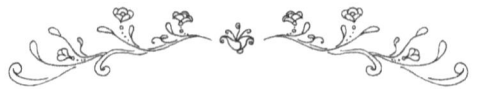

"Wine" and Cheese Rice Pudding
4, 3/4 cup servings - 303 calories each

32 ounces	unsweetened 100% white grape juice
2 tsp	cornstarch
1 cup	Arborio rice
1 Tbsp	honey
2 tsp	vanilla extract
1/4 tsp	cinnamon
1/2 cup	fat-free ricotta cheese

In a medium size sauce pot, whisk the grape juice and cornstarch together. Bring to a boil. Reduce heat and simmer 45 minutes. The juice should reduce to approximately 1-1/2 cups.

Meanwhile, in a separate, medium size sauce pot, combine the rice and 2 cups of water. Bring to a boil, reduce heat and simmer, uncovered, 10 minutes. Add 1-1/2 cups of the reduced grape juice, the honey and vanilla. Bring back to a boil, reduce heat and gently simmer, uncovered, stirring occasionally, 10 minutes.

Remove from heat and add the cinnamon and ricotta. Mix well. Set aside 10 minutes. Transfer to a bowl. Cover and refrigerate until serving time.

Refrigerate any unused "wine". It is delicious warmed and poured over oatmeal, fresh fruit or plain fat-free yogurt.

ENJOY!

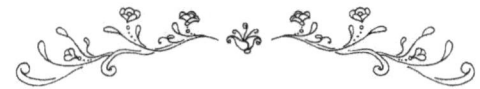

Peanutty Chocolate Covered Banana Cream Parfait
2 servings - 194 calories each

2 ounces	fat-free cream cheese, softened
1 Tbsp	peanut butter, creamy or chunky
2 Tbsp	fat-free vanilla yogurt
1 tsp	mini semi-sweet chocolate chips
1	banana, sliced
2 Tbsp	fat-free non dairy whipped topping

Add the cream cheese, peanut butter and yogurt to a food processor bowl or blender. Process to thoroughly combine. Fold in the chocolate chips.

Make parfaits by spooning alternate layers of banana slices and the cream cheese mixture, dividing both evenly between the 2 servings. Top each with 1 Tbsp of whipped topping.

ENJOY!

Strawberries Italiano
2 servings - 71 calories each

2 cups	strawberries (approx. 10), cored and coarsely chopped
2 tsp	honey
1 tsp	balsamic vinegar
3	fresh basil leaves, stems removed and thinly sliced

In a medium bowl, stir the strawberries and honey together well. Add the balsamic and basil and mix well. Set aside at room temperature 1 hour to macerate.

Stir again, cover and refrigerate 1 hour before using.

Crushed rosemary can be substituted for the fresh basil. Use 1/4 tsp.

Serving Suggestions:
Serve in a bowl topped with fat-free non dairy whipped topping.

Spoon over fat-free yogurt (either regular or frozen), fat-free cottage cheese or angel food cake.

ENJOY!

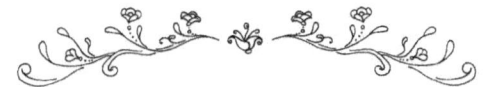

Strawberries and Cream
2 servings - 80 calories each

14	strawberries, cored and sliced
1/8 tsp	ground ginger
1 tsp	dried mint leaves
1 tsp	vanilla extract
4 Tbsp	fat-free non dairy whipped topping
1 tsp	mini semi-sweet chocolate chips

In a medium bowl, combine strawberries, ginger, mint and vanilla. Mix well, crushing the strawberries slightly as you mix. Set aside.

In a separate smaller bowl, combine the whipped topping and chocolate chips. Stir together gently.

Serve the strawberries topped with the whipped topping mixture, dividing them both equally between the two servings.

ENJOY!

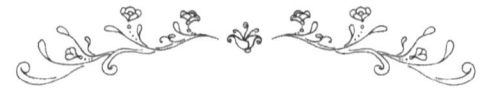

Four Easy, Delicious Fresh Fruit Desserts
<u>2 servings each</u>

Dessert 1-125 calories each
1/2 cup water
2 small or 1 large peach, chopped
8 strawberries, stemmed, chopped
1/4 cup Special K Vanilla Almond cereal, crushed
4 Tbsp fat-free non dairy whipped topping

Dessert 2-169 calories each
1/2 cup water
2 medium apples, cored, diced
20 seedless red or black grapes, halved
1/4 tsp ground cinnamon
1/4 cup Special K Vanilla Almond cereal, crushed
4 Tbsp fat-free non dairy whipped topping

Dessert 3-162 calories each
1/2 cup water
1 banana, sliced
20 strawberries, stemmed, chopped
2 tsp mini semi-sweet chocolate chips
4 Tbsp fat-free non dairy whipped topping

Dessert 4-173 calories each
1/2 cup water
2 cups fresh pineapple, diced
1 medium navel orange, peeled, diced
1/4 cup shredded coconut
4 Tbsp fat-free non dairy whipped topping

Preheat oven to 325 degrees. Pour 1/4 cup water into each of 2 oven-proof ramekin or individual serving dishes.

In a medium size mixing bowl, combine the fruits and cinnamon, if called for. Mix well. Pour into ramekins, dividing it equally between the 2. Top each with half of the cereal or chocolate chips or coconut. Bake for 30 to 35 minutes until fruit is tender and bubbly.

Dollop 2 Tbsp of whipped topping on each.

ENJOY!

Mocha "Latte"
1 serving - 35 calories each

1 package	diet hot chocolate powder mix
3/4 tsp	instant coffee
8 ounces	hot water
1 Tbsp	fat-free non dairy whipped topping

Spoon hot chocolate mix and instant coffee into a mug. Add hot water and stir until powder and coffee are dissolved. Top with whipped topping.

ENJOY!

In Conclusion

"How did you do it?" was the question I heard dozens of times, especially from people I hadn't seen for a long time. I wish my answer to them and to you would be that I had discovered a pill, without deadly side effects we could take once a day to melt the pounds off while we sleep. In lieu of that, I sincerely hope the information in this little book will inspire and motivate you to develop your own personal program that will result in a long-term, healthier lifestyle.

www.ingramcontent.com/pod-product-compliance
Lightning Source LLC
Chambersburg PA
CBHW072259290526
45794CB00002B/513